The "I Have a Life"
Guide to Baby's 1st Year

Get Through Your Baby's First Twelve Months—
Without Losing Your Life—Or Your Mind!

Edited by Indi Zeleny

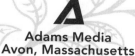

Adams Media
Avon, Massachusetts

Published by Adams Media,
an F+W Publications Company
57 Littlefield Street
Avon, MA 02322
www.adamsmedia.com

ISBN 10: 1-59869-087-6
ISBN 13: 978-1-59869-087-3
Printed in the United States of America.
J I H G F E D C B A

Library of Congress Cataloging
in Publication Data
The "I have a life" guide to baby's 1st year / edited by Indi Zeleny.
p.   cm.
ISBN-13: 978-1-59869-087-3
ISBN-10: 1-59869-087-6
1. Infants–Care. 2. Mother and infant. 3. Parenting. I. Zeleny, Indi. II. Title: "I have a life" guide to baby's first year.
HQ774.I43 2007
649'.122--dc22
2006028417

This book is available at quantity discounts for bulk purchases. For information, please call 1-800-289-0963.

This publication is designed to provide accurate and authoritative information with regard to the subject matter covered. It is sold with the understanding that the publisher is not engaged in rendering legal, accounting, or other professional advice. If legal advice or other expert assistance is required, the services of a competent professional person should be sought.

—From a *Declaration of Principles* jointly adopted by a Committee of the American Bar Association and a Committee of Publishers and Associations

Contains portions of material adapted or abridged from *The Everything® Baby's First Year Book* by Tekla S. Nee ©1997, F+W Publications, Inc.; *The Everything® Mother's First Year Book* by Robin Elise Weiss, ©2005, F+W Publications, Inc.; *The Everything® Breastfeeding Book* by Suzanne Fredregill and Ray Fredregill, ©2002, F+W Publications, Inc.; *The Everything® Get Your Baby to Sleep Book* by Cynthia McGregor, ©2005, F+W Publications, Inc.; *The Everything® Father's First Year Book* by Vincent Iannelli, M.D., ©2005, F+W Publications, Inc.; *The Everything® Baby's First Food Book,* by Janet Mason Tarlov, ©2001, F+W Publications, Inc.

Acknowledgments

Special thanks to:

My amazing mom's group who joined forces when our first children were infants: Rachel Conable, Sara Hapner, Thais Lee, Kim Locke, Maria Nye, Marilyn Radojcich, Erin Ramsden, and Elizabeth Sporleder. We've shared five breathtaking, inspirational, and educational years and we're still going strong!

New moms Julie Cole and Tanya Fadem, with whom I've shared uncountable moments in my second child's first year; wise mamas Krista Holt, Michele Chaney, and Cindy Schroeder; and the wonderful families and teachers at Parents Place in Pacific Grove, California.

Paula Munier, who has been and always will be a catalyst in my life.

My mother, Pim Chavasant, for her immeasurable love and support for our family.

And most of all, my longtime partner Randy, without whom I couldn't have survived or thrived during this great parenting adventure. And to my young daughter and son, who have exploded the doors off our lives—in a good way.

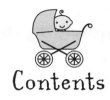

Contents

Introduction

*T*he *"I Have a Life" Guide to Baby's 1ˢᵗ Year*. Sounds like an oxymoron, doesn't it? Who has a new baby *and* a life? Well, I'm here to tell you that you will have a life, albeit a considerably changed life that will range from somewhat similar to totally unrecognizable from its former incarnation—but it is your very own new life, and there's much you can do to send it in the directions you'd like.

This life will be more challenging, but more rewarding, too. The trick is to ease through the learning curve and stay focused, never forgetting the wonderful reason behind this zany first year: your baby. What you're going for is normalization, finding your new normal, while keeping your sense of adventure—and your sense of humor—intact.

There's a school of thought that goes something like this: In the months after you have a baby, you're resigned to life at home in your pajamas, frumpy and overweight, watching soap operas while bouncing a fussy infant on your knee. The good news is that it ain't necessarily so. With admittedly more energy and effort than before, you can still have a life both inside and outside the home, either with baby in tow or with baby safely in the arms of a trusted caregiver.

You need to approach life as an adventure now, an adventure because you must always consider this little person's needs while you engage in your activities, whether you have returned to work or are simply out in the world, shopping, traveling, exercising, and socializing. And this, my new mom, changes everything.

This guide focuses on the topics of most concern to new mothers regarding "having a life": sleep, support, getting out and about with baby, going back to work or staying home, and caregivers. The focus is self-preservation: taking care of you so that you may better care for your child.

We also cover the crucial baby basics to simplify your transition into motherhood and to keep you from having to reinvent the wheel. Peppered throughout are "Smart Mama Tricks" and "Take Care of You" tips to save your sanity and help you through your day—and year.

While we're talking tips, take a tip from the flight attendants: Place the oxygen mask over your nose and mouth before placing it over your child's. If Mommy is exhausted, worn out, and, dare I say it, semi-comatose, how will she ever be able to look after her offspring? You'll find that parenting in this first year is a balancing act, a juggling act, even a three-ring circus, where you at times will play all of the roles—ringmaster, clown, tightrope walker, animal tamer, audience, and participant. But oh what a show, oh what a thrill, and oh what a ride it is!

–Indi Zeleny

Chapter 1

Hello, Baby!

"Giving birth is little more than a set of muscular contractions granting passage of a child. Then the mother is born," wrote Erma Bombeck. Your body and mind are reeling from the birth experience, but this is perfectly normal and okay. The medical staff is busy cleaning and/or stitching you up and perhaps washing the baby, as well. You may be on the high of all highs, or you may feel like you've been run over by a truck—probably a little of both.

Getting to Know You

As you gaze at this tiny infant in your arms, you'll be feeling any combination of emotions: love, fear, joy, relief. Don't worry if you don't have an instant, overwhelming love for your baby. Some moms do, and some moms don't. It can take a little while to get used to your new baby and your new role in life. Try to rest, recuperate, and go with the flow.

Never fear the FLK (Funky-Looking Kid). Fact is, just about every newborn is funky-looking. On arrival, your baby may have:

- Head molding (a conehead, from squeezing through the birth canal)
- Caput (a swelling on the head from fluid squeezed into the scalp)

- Swollen eyelids
- Flattened nose
- Floppy ears
- Fine body hair

- Swollen breasts
- Swollen labia or scrotum
- Peeling skin
- Bluish hands or feet

Your doctor will probably tell you these are normal side effects of birth, and as long as your baby is healthy—don't worry about them!

The point is here, that you did it! You brought a baby into the world and should be elated and proud of yourself!

 Smart Mama Tricks: Bonding Time

Health concerns notwithstanding, baby care such as bathing, weighing, and eye ointment can wait for an hour or two, giving you these precious first moments to cuddle and bond with your baby. Just ask the nurses to wait, or remember to request this in your birth plan ahead of time.

Uh, Waiter?

Of course, you'll try to nurse the baby in the first hour or so, if you feel up for it. But this "food" section is about you. You've just done the physical equivalent of running a marathon, and odds are you're ravenous. Ask the nearest nurse for food and drink. You'll need to keep your energy and calories up for the days and nights ahead and for creating breastmilk.

Somewhere in the hospital room there's a menu. Find it. Check off as many boxes as the staff will allow. If you happened to deliver at an off-hour for food service, send a friend or family member for takeout. If you thought ahead and brought your own snack, by all means, break it out.

Aches & Pains

You will hurt. You don't push something as big as a newborn baby out of as narrow a passage as your vagina without incurring some damage. You may have experienced a natural tear or had an episiotomy, and the stitches in your perineum may pull and itch. You may have gotten through with nary a stitch but have bruised labia. And you may have aches and pains where you never expected them, from your thigh muscles, if you labored standing, to your chest muscles, if you had a hard time pushing. Your tailbone may hurt. You may have hemorrhoids, swollen veins around the rectum that are typically caused by pressure, such as carrying and pushing out a baby.

♡ Take Care of You: **Hemorrhoid Rx**

Hemorrhoids can make having a bowel movement or even sitting down extremely uncomfortable. To find relief, avoid constipation by drinking lots of water and eating fruits and vegetables or by taking a stool softener; soak in a warm bath or sitz bath; and use Tucks pads or witch hazel.

You will also bleed—more than you ever imagined—and that's normal. (But if you're still soaking a thick maternity pad every hour after the first three hours you should alert the nurse or, if you're at home, call your doctor or midwife.) You may have bruises on your face and chest. You may be sweating, as your body sheds the extra fluids it stored during pregnancy. You also may have some odd symptoms—moms have reported itchy rashes that can appear anywhere on the body.

♡ Take Care of You: Place a Guard at the Gate

Many a new mom will casually invite the whole world over to visit her and the baby at the hospital—before she has actually given birth. After the birth, exhausted, emotional, and just wanting some sleep and alone time with close family, you may change your mind. If this occurs, tell the nurses. They can politely inform visitors that the new mommy needs to rest. Later on, if you'd like, you can plead ignorance.

If you had an epidural, you may later have a sore spot in your back where the needle entered. If a catheter was inserted, you may have soreness or a numb feeling in your urethra, compounding your difficulty urinating.

Post C-Section

After a cesarean birth, when the numbness or general anesthesia wears off, you'll feel the most pain at the incision site. Trapped gas that was created when your digestive system was slowed by anesthesia and other drugs can exacerbate this. You can reduce gas pains by getting up and moving as soon as your doctor gives the okay (shuffling slowly down the hospital hall counts, so don't try to do too much). Pressing a pillow against your incision as you climb out of bed can reduce the pain of getting up and moving.

If you have a negative birth experience for whatever reason, you should express this to someone you trust who can validate your feelings. Just because you aren't pleased with your birth experience doesn't mean you don't love your baby. If you have an emergency cesarean, you are six times more likely to experience depression after giving birth. Don't ignore these feelings, or you could find yourself deep in postpartum depression.

Pain Meds

Talk with your doctor about pain-relief options, particularly if you are breastfeeding. Ask the nursing staff if they have a copy of *Medications and Mother's Milk: A Manual of Lactational Pharmacology*, by Thomas W. Hale, Ph.D., a breastfeeding/drug interaction bible. This easy-to-understand tome assigns each medication a lactation risk category, from "safest" to "contraindicated."

The Nurse Is Your Friend

You are the mommy. That means you're the boss. You are also the consumer who is paying for your healthcare services (or hopefully your insurance is), so ask for what you need. Nurses can provide several things for your comfort, including:

- Extra pillows (tuck these behind your back, under your arms, wherever you need for comfort during breastfeeding)
- Topical anesthetic or witch hazel pads (place these cooling pads on top of the sanitary pads, over your perineum)
- More sanitary pads
- A sitz bath
- Stool softener
- Ice, ice, and more ice
- Food and juice and water

And don't think the nurse is the only one at your beck and call! Have Dad do diaper duty, dressing and undressing, swaddling, holding, and carrying your newborn as much as possible while in the hospital. He can learn from the nurses, too, and be all the more prepared to help out once you arrive home. If you had a home birth, Dad can learn from the midwife and her assistants.

Chances are, you will have several different nurses during your stay. They will trot in and out of your room seemingly every twenty minutes, changing your bedding, checking your sutures, if any, and your general healing down there, waking you to take your blood pressure, pulse rate, and temperature just five minutes after you've fallen asleep, checking that your uterus is returning to normal size, and, of course, checking on your newborn.

The checking-on-the-baby part can be reassuring, but the revolving door that keeps you awake after you've already been sleepless forever can become, at the very least, annoying. Tell the nurses how tired you are. Beg them to help you get a little more sleep. They must monitor your vitals, but they will help you get some shut-eye if they can.

Smart Mama Tricks: Rectal Thermometer 101

Ask a nurse to show you how to take your baby's rectal temperature. Then try it yourself on your infant, with the nurse at your side. You don't want to attempt it for the first time alone at home on a crying, sick baby.

Voyage to the Bathroom

One of the nurses' most critical tasks is to make sure that you urinate. They will harass you about urinating at a time when you wish they would leave you alone. They will get clearly irritated, if not hostile, if you forgetfully urinate and flush the toilet without telling anyone. Peeing may be the last thing in the world you want to do, but you have to—if you don't, you can endanger your life.

The first trip to the bathroom will probably not be something you are looking forward to. It may feel fine, or it may hurt because your urethra was banged up during the birth. You may also find that once you get there you simply can't pee, either from fear of pain or because of damage to your perineum. You can help to avoid this burning feeling by spraying warm water onto your perineum (the hospital should give you a "peri-bottle" for this purpose) while you urinate.

♡ Take Care of You: I'll Have Mine to Go

When you're preparing to leave the hospital, ask for extra painkillers, stool softeners, and sanitary pads if you think you'll need them, and pack your peri-bottles and sitz bath to take home with you.

The first bowel movement can also be scary; your muscles relaxed during the birth and you have to push a lot harder to get a bowel movement out. After a birth the idea of doing anything like pushing seems crazy, and pushing against stitches—if you have them—does hurt. This is where stool softeners come in handy.

The Expedition Home

If this is your first baby, you may hesitate to leave the security of your hospital room. After all, the nurses and doctors have cared for you and your newborn around the clock. Now you're supposed to take this helpless infant out into the real world—into a moving vehicle, possibly at highway speeds, all the way home—and then take total responsibility for him from here on out? No wonder you're nervous. But rest assured; you'll do just fine.

Most insurance covers a forty-eight-hour hospital stay for a vaginal birth, longer for a cesarean birth. Even if this is your second or third baby and you're feeling confident, consider staying at the hospital for the full allotted time. Remember: Once you get home, household chores and sibling requirements will likely overtake you no matter how helpful your partner and family may be.

 Smart Mama Tricks: **Car-Seat Check**

Car seats have always been hard to use, and most experts estimate that 85 percent of parents use them incorrectly. There are trained professionals who can evaluate your car seat and its installation for you. Find them at www.seatcheck.org or 1-866-SEAT-CHECK. If you can, take advantage of this before the birth of your baby.

In addition to a car seat, remember to bring a blanket to shield your baby from rain or sun. You may want to ride in the backseat with your baby during the first car trip or two to watch and comfort him—and to set your mind at ease. You may find that you see the world differently once your baby is riding in your car. Suddenly it seems like every vehicle is pointed directly at yours and every driver is an inconsiderate lunatic. Don't they realize that there is a *baby* in your car? These initial fears are normal and will fade in time.

Chapter 2

Back in the Nest

If this is your first baby, the first several days home may feel less like home and more like you've landed on another planet. There's an alien creature in your house and, well, it's taking over. Give it a little more time while you heal and get accustomed to the little person in your life. You may be wondering whether or not you are really prepared for this. Take a deep breath and let the New World Order begin.

Your New-Life Mottos

Here are four. You'll come up with more over the course of a year.

- **Be Prepared:** Have a full complement of diapers, wipes, blankets, food and drink (for you) at the ready where and when you need them. Post the numbers for your pediatrician, doctor or midwife, and nurse's hotline by the phone. You have license to rearrange the house to fit your current needs.
- **Be Flexible:** Plans change according to your baby's whims, hunger, and sleep habits. At the very least, you won't arrive anywhere on time. Just as you head out the front door, your baby will invariably have a blow-out poopy diaper that you'll have to change.

- **Trust Your Instincts:** If something really worries you, it's probably serious enough to warrant action or at least a closer look. If your baby looks "off" and really isn't herself, but you don't know what's wrong, it's time to call the pediatrician. If you're wondering whether your four-month-old might be able to roll along the floor over to the dresser on the other side of the room and reach her chubby arm behind it and grab the electrical cord, bank on it and fix it. Most often, Mother really does know best.
- **Memorize and repeat, "This too will pass":** When things get tough, really tough, and you're not sure you can make it through this latest phase in your (or your baby's) life, know that things will change. When life seems hard, it will get better. When life is wonderful, enjoy it to the fullest, because it too will change at some point. Change is the only constant. You need to go with the flow.

Smart Mama Tricks: **Mum's the Word**

Don't correct your partner when he changes a diaper or attempts to comfort your crying baby. It's vital that your mate bond with your baby, too. You're not just nurturing a child; you're nurturing a family.

If you still have perineal pain or if your hemorrhoids still hurt, continue to use your peri-bottle and your Tucks pads. To help relieve both of these conditions, run a shallow bath or use your sitz bath.

Healing at Home

Your hormone levels are shifting and adjusting, you're healing, you're up at all hours, you're excited and maybe you're nervous, too. Simply put, you're tired. Your job is to rest and recuperate from labor and delivery.

Rest, Rest, Then Rest Some More

Although babies sleep about sixteen-and-a-half hours a day during the first week of life, and maybe even more during the first few days, baby's sleep time will rarely seem to coincide with yours. You will hear this again and again: Sleep when the baby sleeps. At first, this might seem impossible, given that you're used to sleeping only once every twenty-four hours, preferably for at least an eight-hour stretch. Know that it will be a few weeks or months before your infant gets into a regular pattern of sleeping more at night. Until then, she probably will sleep and eat on regular two- to four-hour cycles. (Note: If your baby does sleep most of the day away and rarely cries or fusses, check with your pediatrician. What you may think is great baby behavior could be a sign of illness. Periods of wakefulness or distress in babies are common and completely healthy.)

Whatever the case may be, try to temporarily alter your sleep pattern so that you sleep at the same time as your infant, day or night. You will be tempted—in truth, compelled—to "get things done" while your baby naps. Fact is, dishes can wait. Laundry can wait. You cannot wait. You must get sleep or you will not function, and you must function well in order to take care of your infant.

Accept Help—and Live in Your Jammies!

People will ask what they can do for you. Housecleaning, cooking, and laundry top the list. Perhaps your partner, mother, or your experienced best friend can hold the baby while you catch some z's.

One way to ensure that you do rest and spend time alone with your baby is to stay in your nightgown and robe. First of all, it reminds you—and everyone else—that the most important thing you can do for yourself at this point is rest and let other people take care of you. You're a lot less likely to want to do chores around the house or run an errand if you're in your nightgown, and people (like your partner) are less likely to expect you to do anything more than feed your baby.

♡ Take Care of You: **The Food Train**

Have a good friend or family member organize a food train as soon as the baby is born. Friends and relatives sign up for one evening each where they'll drop off a dinner for your family. When you factor in leftovers, you might not have to cook for weeks. Note: Inform visitors ahead of time that it is just a food drop-off, not a full-fledged visit. Set a time limit, then politely excuse yourself.

Feeding the Family

Hopefully, you've planned ahead and cooked and frozen a couple of weeks' worth of nutritious meals. Restaurant takeout is your friend. Collect your favorite local restaurants' to-go menus and have them at the ready. Many cities have some form of takeout delivery service that covers a range of restaurants for one delivery fee.

If your partner can cook, so much the better for you. When you must do the cooking, double the recipe and freeze half for another day.

Feeding You

If you're nursing, you need 500 calories a day more than when you were pregnant just to maintain your weight. Include eight eight-ounce glasses of noncaffeinated fluid. If you drink when you're thirsty and your urine is light in color, you know your fluid intake is adequate. You'll quickly learn that you shouldn't go far without bringing a drink and a snack along.

Early Baby Care

In the first days, you'll spend most of your time holding, nursing, bonding with, and diapering your baby. You'll spend countless hours just memorizing her face and gazing at her precious little fingers and toes. Before you know it, you're ready to try something a bit more advanced, say, bathing and nail trimming.

Body Basics

Of course, your infant's entire body is worthy of intense adoration and scrutiny, but these three places tend to raise the most questions:

- **The Floppy Head:** Always support baby's head and neck when lifting, carrying, or turning her over. Her poor head control and lack of strong neck muscles can cause her head to quickly fall or flop backward, which can hurt her. (Note: Never, ever shake a baby. Even a brief episode of shaking for five or ten seconds can cause brain damage or even death.)
- **The Soft Spot:** Your baby's soft spot, or fontanel, is where the different plates of her skull come together. Although this part of her head isn't protected by bone, it is still fairly tough and is not easy to push through during the regular day-to-day tasks that you do to take care of her. Don't worry too much about the soft spot when you put on your baby's hat, brush or wash her hair, or simply pat her head—but don't push directly on her soft spot.
- **The Stump:** First, keep baby's umbilical-cord stump dry—no real baths until it falls off. Until then, just continue to give her sponge baths when necessary. It also helps to leave the cord exposed to the air by not covering it with a diaper or clothes. Some doctors recommend swabbing the base of the cord with a little rubbing alcohol; others think it prolongs the time it takes for the stump to fall off. Call your pediatrician if your child develops an infection of the umbilical-cord stump. Signs can include a persistent, foul-smelling discharge and redness around the belly button.

Bathing Beauty

Bath time is easy for most of the first month until your baby's umbilical cord comes off, because she will only need a sponge bath a few times a week. Expect that she won't like these early baths, though.

The Sponge Bath

First, get everything ready beforehand. Here's what you'll need:

- A bath thermometer
- A basin filled with warm water and a mild soap
- Two or more washcloths for cleaning different areas of the body (e.g., one for her bottom and one for her face)
- A cup of warm water or your spray peri-bottle from the hospital, for rinsing
- A soft surface to place your baby on, such as the bed or kitchen counter with another towel on it
- A diaper and clean clothes

Once you're ready, make sure the room is warm and free from drafts. Ensure that the water is not too hot—about 90 degrees Fahrenheit is safe. Undress your baby and wrap her in a towel. Place her on the soft surface you have chosen and gently wash (patting, not scrubbing) each part of her body with the washcloth you have dipped in the basin of soapy water.

Pay special attention to all the creases around her neck, which may be filled with gunk. With a newborn, this gunk is likely skin cells sloughing off or residue from spit-up milk (affectionately known in some circles as "neck cheese"). Of course, never leave baby unattended on a high place and always keep at least one hand on her body, just like you would on a changing table. Rinse her off when you're done and wrap her in another towel to get dry.

Smart Mama Tricks: **Just Right**

Always test the water temperature before putting your baby in the tub. A bath thermometer works best (90 degrees Fahrenheit). Otherwise, use the inside of your wrist or your elbow rather than your fingers to judge. Aim for comfortably warm, not hot.

The Full Bath

Once the cord has fallen off, you may prepare for baby's first bath. You can bathe your infant by holding her in a small baby bathtub or by holding her with you in the full-size bathtub. Whichever method you choose, again have everything you need in arm's reach before you start the bathing process. A word to the wise: Wet babies are slippery.

Never leave baby unsupervised in the tub for even a few seconds. A baby can drown in that much time. Don't assume that a bath ring or seat will be enough to keep your baby safe—these are meant to make bath time easier, not provide supervision, and have been known to tip over. Have your cordless phone nearby or, better yet, don't answer the phone during bath time.

You'll need the same supplies as with a sponge bath, substituting the baby bathtub or your own bathtub for the basin of water. It helps to have another adult to assist the first few times while you get used to the process.

If you use the baby bathtub, try to find a safe place, such as a countertop, where you can work at a height that is comfortable for your back. Placing the little tub inside your bathtub may seem easier as far as cleanup is concerned, but it can put a real strain on your body to bend over so far. Remember to support her head and neck and hold most of her body just above the small amount of soapy water that you put in the baby tub. You will then wash and rinse her with a washcloth and warm water.

 Smart Mama Tricks: **Skip the Everyday Bath**

Infants don't get dirty the way young children do and only need the occasional baths to keep their skin healthy. Forgo the daily bath until your baby starts crawling on the floor. Bathing two or three times a week, in addition to thorough cleansing after feedings and changes, is sufficient for now.

If you bathe together, run the bath slightly cooler than you normally would for yourself (again, use the thermometer to test the water), get into

Back in the Nest

the bath, and have someone hand baby to you. Take special precautions so that you won't slip. Of course, make sure that your baby isn't totally submerged in the water, and always keep at least one hand supporting her head and neck. Cuddle your baby against your chest and neck and help her get used to the tub. Nursing is okay here, as well, and will help baby get used to the bathtub and see it as a comforting place. (Remember that newborns often poop right after nursing!) When you're finished, hand baby back to your helper while you get out of the tub. Gently towel her dry.

Nail Trimming

Infant nail trimming often strikes fear into the new mother's heart. But with the right equipment, proper lighting, and a calm or, better yet, sleeping baby, it's a snap. More important, it saves baby from having to wear those cotton mittens all the time or risk scratching her face with those fast-growing, sharp little talons. Plus, you'll get better at it the more you try, so you may as well get started.

 Smart Mama Tricks: **Clippers or Scissors?**

Trying to decide between clippers and scissors? Try using what you're most comfortable using on your own nails. You'll be more experienced with that implement and less likely to accidentally nick or pinch baby's skin.

Wait until your baby is in a deep sleep. This means her arms and legs flop when lifted and her hand is resting open, not in a fist. Hold the manicure scissors or infant clippers in one hand; with the other, pull the tip of her finger down away from the nail. You should now have better access to the nail, so go ahead and cut—straight across. If you're worried about sharp corners, you can gently file them later. If you do cut your baby, press on the cut and the bleeding will quickly stop.

♡ Take Care of You

Now that baby is all clean and groomed, try taking her for walks in the stroller or sling/front pack. The exercise will improve your mood, the motion will settle your baby own, and everyone you meet will coo at the baby and fuss over you, which can give you an ego boost when you need it most!

If you still can't bring yourself to cut your baby's nails, try using a small piece of an Emory board to gently file them down while she sleeps. Some moms continue to use this method until the baby's fingers grow to a more manageable size.

Chapter 3

For Crying Out Loud

When your baby is born, he typically greets the world with a wail. You'll probably be thrilled to hear that first cry. This may also be the last time you will be happy to hear your baby cry. For the next few years, in fact, you may put a lot of effort into getting your child to *stop* crying. As we all know, all babies cry. So read on to educate yourself about what his crying actually means.

Crybabies

The first few days after birth, your baby may do nothing but sleep, and hardly cry at all. Don't congratulate yourself yet. Although some babies really do cry much less often than others and your infant may well be one of these "ideal" babies, crying doesn't really get going until babies are a few weeks old, then usually peaks at six weeks.

Contrary to popular belief, crying is not your baby's only way to communicate with you. In fact, it is usually his last signal that something is bothering him. Your baby will give other cues (facial expressions, heavy breathing, etc.), and you should learn to recognize these. That way, you'll be better able to respond to your child before he has to cry.

Get the Message

A crying baby is trying to tell you something. He may be trying to communicate that he's hungry, or that he ate too much and his stomach hurts. He may be saying that his diaper is wet and it feels yucky, or that he liked that nice warm wet diaper on him and now that you took it off, he's cold—and mad! He may be saying that he's tired and wants you to rock him to sleep, or that he's bored and wants you to samba dance for his entertainment. He may be saying that he's furious that he can't scoot across the carpet and grab the fireplace tools—in which case he's going to be crying for the next six or seven months (but will probably crawl early). When you first hold your squalling baby in your arms, you won't understand any of this.

 Smart Mama Tricks: **Have a Ball**

Keep a large exercise/labor ball in the house. Hold a fussing baby close against you, or in a sling or front pack, and sit and bounce gently. The motion is more restful for you than pacing back and forth through the house and often lulls the baby to sleep. Be sure to first check your balance on the ball without holding your infant.

Your job is to figure out how to understand your infant's language, because crying is a language. The sooner you figure it out, the sooner you'll spend more time listening to your baby coo and babble and less time listening to him shriek.

What you shouldn't be doing, at this point, is trying to teach your baby patience. Don't make him wait while you finish unloading the dishwasher, for example. In fact, the faster you respond to his cries, the better: It's easier to calm a baby who has just started crying, before it escalates into hysteria.

Unspoiled

Today, almost all child-rearing experts agree that you should hold and soothe your baby when he cries. Responding to your baby when he's asking for your help will lay the foundation for a close and trusting relationship. In fact, instinctively, you will want to pick up your baby when he cries; it seems to be hard-wired into moms, and probably not without reason.

Hold Me

So how much holding is too much? Really, you can't overdo it. Parents who practice "attachment parenting" even advocate that your baby be in close contact with you for most of the time. Attachment parents believe that babies are meant to be carried. In some cultures, babies are carried as much as 90 percent of the time, and they don't cry as much as babies in industrialized countries (who spend more of their time alone). In fact, researchers have confirmed that extra carrying results in dramatic reductions in crying. If you don't want your baby to let out more than a whimper once in a while, don't put him down.

This isn't as onerous as it may seem. With such options as front packs and slings, and backpacks for older babies, your child can be "worn" comfortably for hours, leaving your hands free to do other things. (For more on baby carriers, see Chapter 11, Mobile Mom.)

Instead of worrying about whether or not you will spoil your baby, trust your instincts and hold him when it seems right.

Fuss-Busters

When your baby cries, try not to get frustrated. Instead, be a problem solver. Assess the situation by asking yourself questions. Could your baby be hungry? Is he tired? Does he need to be changed? In some cases, your baby will be asking you simply for a change of environment. For instance, if he is in a swing, moving him to a calmer place—like a blanket on the floor—might help him relax. If you are in a noisy room, try moving him to a quieter area. If you're inside, step out-of-doors.

Get a Move On

When you've ensured that baby is not hungry, wet, hot, or tired—or perhaps you know he's tired but is having trouble falling asleep—movement can help. Rock with him in your glider or rocking chair, or stand up and do the tried-and-true rhythmic, knee-bending, bouncy walks. Try carrying your baby in a sling or a front pack and going for a walk—around the house or around the block. Most baby stores sell battery-operated baby swings that gently rock back and forth, and some parents swear by these. Other babies loathe them. See if you can have your baby test-drive a friend's swing before you buy one of your own.

Distractions

Play different kinds of music to catch his interest. If classical doesn't work, reggae might. Or give your baby something interesting to look at: a plant, a mobile, or even a brightly patterned tablecloth. Describe what you're looking at and keep talking softly.

Swaddling

In the first few weeks, some babies feel more secure, and are less likely to fuss, when wrapped snuggly. Swaddling will contain his flailing arms and legs, which may be startling him, and calm him down. (Other babies hate this and will quickly let you know.) Baby does need time to exercise his limbs, so swaddle only at night. Remember that the baby will be warmer wrapped in the blanket, so dress him accordingly or lower the temperature in the room.

HOW TO SWADDLE AN INFANT:

1. Position square blanket like a diamond; fold the top corner down.
2. Lay your baby on his back on the blanket, the top corner just above his neck. Tuck one arm down and fold the blanket around his body and behind his back.
3. Fold up the bottom part of the blanket, folding down any excess that would be covering his face.
4. Tuck the other arm down and fold the remaining corner of the blanket around his body and behind his back.

Could It Be Colic?

Popular wisdom says that if you have to ask, it's not colic—that truly colicky infants leave no doubt in their parents' minds. Colic basically means you have a baby that cries a lot with seemingly no rational cause, and he doesn't respond, at least for very long, to soothing. This may mean a baby is just venting at the end of a long day. But if the crying goes on for hours every day, at roughly the same time, several days a week, then you can feel justified in calling it colic. Some pediatricians use the Rule of Three to diagnose colic: crying for no apparent physical reason for three hours a day, three days a week, for three weeks. By this definition, one out of five babies may have colic.

♡ Take Care of You: Don't Stop Breastfeeding

Just because your baby is fussy doesn't necessarily mean that something is wrong with his breastfeeding, that he isn't getting enough to eat, or that you should switch to formula. This is almost never helpful. Talk to your pediatrician or a lactation consultant before you stop nursing your fussy baby.

After beginning at about two to three weeks of age, colic usually reaches its peak at six weeks and then gradually improves over the next month or two. Generally, it stops somewhere around the three-month mark.

If you have a baby who cries excessively, see your pediatrician for an evaluation before you simply decide that you have a fussy baby. Although there's usually nothing to worry about, medical conditions that lead to such excessive crying can be serious and you should check it out. At the same time, you also don't want to put your baby through a lot of unnecessary tests or treatments.

♡ Take Care of You: Know When to Say When

When your baby cries on and on for seemingly no reason at all, you've tried every trick you know to no avail, and you feel yourself losing it, hand your baby off to someone else, if possible. Now you can calm down, and the change may distract baby from his carrying on. Or put your little one someplace safe, like in his car seat on the floor or in his crib, and briefly leave the room to regain your composure. Call 911 if you need to. Losing control can have dangerous repercussions.

By the time you get through three or four dietary changes for the mom (if you're breastfeeding) or formula changes for the baby (if you aren't), two or three medicines for reflux, and an upper GI, your baby with colic will probably already have reached his peak time of crying and will be getting better on his own. Whether or not there is a medical cause for your baby's crying that needs attention, try different ways to soothe your baby and ease his crying.

Be There Now

Meanwhile, if medical conditions have been ruled out, nothing you do seems to affect the crying, and you are *not* at your wit's end, consider just holding your baby while he cries. (And enlist your partner, your relatives, and your friends to hold him, too.) You're sending the message that you'll be there through the best of times and the worst of times. To calm yourself during this process, try giving the baby permission to cry. Sounds funky perhaps, but if you calmly repeat to your infant, "It's okay to cry" or "Go ahead and let it out. Just cry, cry, cry," it may help you to accept the whole situation. Or sing a song. Even if it doesn't seem to help the baby, it's hard for you to lose your temper when you are singing "Merrily, merrily, merrily, merrily, life is but a dream." Finally, know that this particular crying jag will end—likely with an exhausted, sleeping baby. And someday soon, the whole crying phase will be a distant memory.

Chapter 4

Breastfeeding

You have a big choice to make. Sure, you've been making decision after decision since this whole roller coaster of babymaking, pregnancy, and childbirth started. But this is one of the biggies. Not only is breastfeeding healthful for your child and for you, it will also make your new life with baby much easier.

Why Breast Is Best

For at least your baby's first six months of life, eating means milk—breastmilk or infant formula. More than 95 percent of mothers are physically capable of breastfeeding. If you can, you should. Here's why: Human milk is designed as the perfect food for infants. It contains elements that researchers are only beginning to discover. And there are hundreds of ingredients identified in breastmilk that are missing from infant formula. However, even if every ingredient in human milk could be duplicated, breastmilk would still have significant advantages over formula.

The Many Benefits of Breastfeeding

Here are a few more reasons why breastfeeding is the best option for feeding your baby:

- Breastmilk provides the exact nourishment your baby needs at each stage of her development from birth to weaning, adjusting in subtle ways as your baby matures.
- Colostrum, the yellowish fluid produced in the first few days, provides babies with antibodies to protect them from the germs they are encountering.
- Breastmilk contains antibodies important for bolstering your baby's developing immune system.
- Breastmilk contains all of the right enzymes, designed specifically for the human digestive tract, to help babies efficiently absorb the milk's nutrients with a minimum of discomfort.
- Breastmilk contains literally thousands of nutrients designed by nature for human babies. Many of these nutrients and their beneficial properties have yet to be identified.
- Studies show fewer illnesses and more contented dispositions in babies who are breastfed.
- Studies have found up to a ten-point IQ advantage in breastfed children.
- Breastfeeding exercises baby's entire mouth (as opposed to bottle feeding, which exercises only the front). These sucking movements help breastfed babies develop larger nasal space and better jaw alignment, which lowers risk of snoring, sleep apnea, and orthodontic work later in life.

- Hormones released during lactation in the first days and weeks following delivery help the mother's uterus contract back to its normal size more quickly, hastening recovery.
- Many women who breastfeed experience a more rapid loss of unwanted weight gained during pregnancy.
- Most mothers find nursing a convenient way to feed their baby, because once a nursing routine is established, a baby can be quickly and easily fed with a minimum of fuss.
- Studies show that breastfed babies are less likely to experience food allergies later in life and may have a lower risk of developing diabetes.
- Increasing evidence indicates that breastfeeding decreases the mother's risk for osteoporosis, as well as uterine, cervical, breast, and ovarian cancer.
- Formula is expensive. If you choose bottle feeding, you can expect to spend over $1,200 annually on formula alone. Costs for nursing a baby include only the additional food consumed by the mother.

Simplicity

Breastfeeding is easy. Most of you will discover this after the initial awkwardness. Others may find that the first few weeks of figuring out how to breastfeed correctly are a challenge. When your breastfed baby is hungry, you pick her up, unsnap your nursing bra or lift up your regular bra, and dinner is served. Once you get the hang of it, you'll probably manage to have a free hand—until it's time to switch to the other side. You can read, dial a telephone, even shop for groceries (online or walking down store aisles) while your baby nurses in a sling.

♡ Take Care of You: **No Periods!**

Many women enjoy time off from their menses for the first six months of breastfeeding. As long as you are exclusively breastfeeding, you're much less likely to become pregnant. With lactational amenorrhea, women enjoy a 98 to 99 percent effective method of birth control. Best of all, it's completely natural.

When your bottle-fed baby is hungry, you have to check the refrigerator or the diaper bag and hope you find a prepared bottle, then possibly warm it up while trying to distract your hungry and increasingly agitated baby. And bottle-feeding is a two-handed operation; you can't do much else while you're holding both the baby and the bottle.

The American Academy of Pediatrics (AAP) recommends:

- Mothers breastfeed for at least the first twelve months of life and as long after as is mutually desired
- Babies breastfeed exclusively for the first six months of life
- Newborns nurse whenever they show signs of hunger
- No supplements—including water or formula—be given to breast-feeding newborns unless there is medical indication

Breastmilk is easier to digest than formula, so breastfed babies rarely get diarrhea or constipation and (this is a biggie) their dirty diapers don't stink. There is an odor, but not a particularly bad one. In fact, the stuff looks kind of like Dijon mustard and smells a bit like buttermilk headed south.

Mellow Mommy

You, too, will reap the rewards of breastfeeding. Skin-to-skin contact and suckling release powerful stress-reducing hormones in your body that relax you and give you a calm, pleasurable feeling. Those same hormones help you to literally fall in love with your newborn.

 Smart Mama Tricks: **The Original Convenience Food**

One of the nicest things about breastfeeding is the convenience. The milk is always the perfect temperature, it's always clean, and you can't forget your breasts when you leave the house.

These hormones also prevent the short-term feeling of sadness some women experience after childbirth. "Baby blues" results from the sudden drop in pregnancy hormones in your body after delivery, and breastfeeding signals your body to release the hormones that prevent those blues. If you breastfeed immediately following birth and wean gradually at a time of your choice, you might avoid the baby blues altogether.

Healthcare Professionals Agree

Again, breastmilk is the best milk for your baby. The American Academy of Pediatrics (AAP), the World Health Organization (WHO), The Association of Women's Health, Obstetric and Neonatal Nursing (AWHONN), the Federation International of Gynecology & Obstetrics (FIGO), the International Confederation of Midwives (ICM), the International Lactation Consultant Association (ILCA), the Women, Infants, and Children Supplemental Program (WIC), and the U.S. Department of Health and Human Services all recommend *exclusive* breastfeeding for at least the first six months.

At the Hospital

Newborns are hardwired for breastfeeding. They can zero in on the darkened bull's-eye of the areola and can see your face clearly while nursing at your breast. Babies nuzzle the nipple aggressively to make it erect for latching onto. They also have the ability to "crawl" to the breast within the first hour after birth and to memorize the smell of your breastmilk.

In your birth plan, you noted that you intended to breastfeed. If you haven't already, now is the time to meet with a lactation consultant—a professional in the art of breastfeeding. Most hospitals have one on staff. They can instruct you in every aspect of breastfeeding and show you how to successfully nurse your baby.

If your baby must stay in the nursery, hospital staff should bring the baby to you for feeding every two to three hours around the clock. If your baby is rooming in with you, which is highly recommended for breastfeeding, the hospital staff will remind you to nurse often. This will increase your milk supply and will also help you retain what you've learned about breastfeeding.

♡ Take Care of You: **Videotape the Proceedings**

If you happen to have a video camera handy, tape the lactation consultant's demonstrations. They'll be invaluable when you go home and are on your own.

Ready, Set, Go!

Your baby has just made her entrance into the world, and, if she's doing fine, your partner or a nurse has placed her on your stomach. You can try to breastfeed her right away if you're up for it, but don't feel like you have to; waiting until you both get your bearings is fine. And even if you're ready, your baby may not be. Don't sweat it. There really is no rush. You'll both probably have a nap in the hours following the birth. Then you'll both wake up ready to tackle this new experience. When your baby is ready for that very first feeding, go ahead and try it.

Hold Everything

You'll probably want to start with the football hold or cradle hold. Sit up in bed, pull up your hospital gown, and settle a pillow on your lap. Make sure your back and elbows are supported; you may need more pillows. Get comfortable. If you have large breasts, tuck a rolled-up wash-cloth or towel under the breast you intend to nurse with to help support it. Then ask the nurse or your partner to hand you the baby.

Smart Mama Tricks: Banish the Binky

Don't use a pacifier until a solid nursing routine is established, if you plan to use one at all. You want your baby to suck on you to encourage and build a strong milk supply.

Unwrap your baby and pull up her T-shirt, if she's wearing one. You want skin to touch skin.

Use pillows to bring her up to the level of your breast. Rotate your baby to face your breast, supporting her head. It's important that when you are chest to breast with your baby, her ear, shoulder, and hip form a straight line.

Docking with the Mothership

Now, for the all-important latch: With the opposite hand, form a C with your thumb and forefinger and cup beneath your breast, like the way you hold a sandwich, only upside down. Bring the baby close to your breast (don't lean down to the baby, that's a sure path to back pain), and lift up your nipple making sure not to cover the areola with your hand.

Tickle the baby's lips with the tip of your nipple. You might tickle her cheek or bottom lip to stimulate her rooting reflex, if needed. Wait until she opens really wide like a yawn, and then, bringing her head to your breast, shove your breast in as far as it will go. If you aren't quick enough, your baby may have only the nipple in her mouth. Use your finger to break the suction, take her off the breast, and try again. You may have to try several times to get this right. Remember, you're both new at this.

♡ Take Care of You: More Help, Please

If you are unclear about anything regarding breastfeeding, ask your nurse or lactation consultant again (if you're at home, your midwife will probably still be there to help). Don't be intimidated by a busy hospital or a buzzing nurse. This is your time. What you learn now can determine your immediate breastfeeding success.

Once she's on, check her position. Her mouth should be covering at least a third of the areola and you should hear sucks and swallows. Don't fuss about whether or not her nose seems to be covered by the breast—if she can't breathe, she'll move. Switch sides when you think your baby has drained the first breast; you won't hear swallowing anymore, or see her jaws or cheeks working. This may take as few as five minutes or longer than twenty or more. Take a burp break when you switch breasts.

How to Break the Latch

Insert your finger into your baby's mouth at the inside cheek to release suction. Hook the nipple and draw it out as you pull your breast away. Baby might try to relatch, but if your hooked finger is covering your nipple, she can't. If you allow your baby to slide off the nipple while she's still creating suction, you'll have sore or cracked nipples. Breaking the latch will be a smooth process once you've tried it a couple of times.

LATCH EVALUATION CHECKLIST

- Does your baby have the entire nipple and at least one inch of the areola in her mouth?
- After your milk lets down, can you hear your baby swallow?
- Does baby follow a "suck, suck, suck, swallow" pattern?
- Can you see noticeable movement in her jaw all the way to her ear (ear wiggling)?
- Is the area at her temple moving?
- Are her lips flanged or everted around the nipple?
- If you hear a clicking sound, that indicates improper latch; break the latch and reposition.
- If you feel pain (excluding the tingling sensation of letdown), break the latch and reposition.
- If your baby is taking in only the nipple, break the latch and reposition.
- If something just doesn't feel right, break the latch and reposition.

Breastfeeding should not be painful. If your baby is positioned on your areola correctly, you should not feel anything more than a slight tug. Pain is often the result of nipple feeding, and continued nipple feeding will lead to cracked or sore nipples and even greater discomfort.

 Smart Mama Tricks: Practice While Pregnant

If you are still pregnant and have a doll available, practice holding positions and the art of bringing baby to breast (not breast to baby). Don't wait until the last minute—breastfeeding is a learned art, and practice makes perfect.

Burping and Spitting

Breastfed babies usually take in less air with their feedings than bottle-fed infants. But all babies need to be burped or they will cry when air bubbles sit in their tummies. Burping should be slow and relatively gentle. You'll find that light patting and rubbing should produce the desired results within a few minutes. As with all the rest of the breastfeeding and burping routines, you will learn to understand what's "normal" for your baby over time.

Breastfeeding and Burping Positions

Try these positions to find what works best for your baby:

- **Over-the-shoulder burping.** Hold baby against your chest with her head over your shoulder. Gently rub or pat her back until she burps.
- **Sitting-upright burping.** Sit baby on your knee and support her with the spread fingers of your hand on her chest. Use the web area of your hand to support her chin. The other hand supports her back as you gently pat her back to burp her.
- **Over-the-lap burping.** Place baby on her tummy and across your lap. Pat or rub her back until she burps. Take care not to bounce your legs as this will upset her tummy and she'll spit up on your shoes.

Although breastfed babies spit up less often than formula-fed infants, you can still expect to have a little of your breastmilk returned to you. Don't be alarmed if your baby occasionally spews. It may look like she spit up her entire meal, but it's often not as much as it appears. Take a tablespoon of water and dump it on the counter. It might look like a lot, but considering your baby is taking in two or more ounces at a single feeding, a tablespoon is a drop in the bucket. However, report any excessive or projectile vomiting to your doctor.

Nursing Tips

While you and your baby are still learning to breastfeed, there are several things you can do to keep things going smoothly:

- Find a comfortable place that will become your nursing nest: a couch, a rocker, or your bed. Use pillows to support your elbows, arms, and back. Use a footrest, a telephone book, or last week's laundry to support your feet.
- Bring the baby to you, instead of moving yourself to the baby.
- Make sure your baby's head is tipped slightly back and her chin is pressed into your breast. It is the movements of her chin and tongue that draw out the milk.
- Keep your wrist straight. Flexing the wrist that is supporting your baby's head may tip her down into a less efficient nursing position, and the strain on your wrist may cause inflammation and pain.
- Nurse at least ten to twelve times a day for the first few weeks—that's an average of every two hours.
- Don't watch the clock; let your baby tell you when she's done.
- Offer one breast first, and when baby is finished, offer the second, alternating the starting lineup at each feeding. (Note that if you have an abundant supply of breastmilk, your baby may fill up completely on just one breast.)
- Vary your nursing position. The baby will press on your breasts differently depending on how she is positioned.
- Try burping when you switch sides and after breastfeeding. But don't worry if your baby doesn't burp; some just don't.

How It All Works

During the first day or two of his life, your baby is nourished not with milk, but with your colostrum, the ideal first food for your infant. When your milk comes in—two to four days after birth—replacing the colostrum, you will know it. Your normally squishy breasts will get bigger than you ever imagined possible and may seem as hard as rocks. Fetch your baby and start nursing, because the longer you wait, the more your breasts will hurt.

 Smart Mama Tricks: Which Side Are We On?

Some clever moms switch a ring back and forth between left and right hands to match the breast that is nursed on first. Try this or come up with your own best way to remember on which side to start the next feeding.

If your breasts are too hard for your baby to latch on to, put a warm washcloth on them for a few minutes or take a shower. You can also massage your milk glands toward your nipple and squeeze out a little milk. If you are still uncomfortable after your baby nurses, put ice on your breasts for a few minutes, or tuck a cold cabbage leaf into your bra for several minutes (don't do this for longer periods of time, as cabbage can reduce your milk supply).

Supply and Demand

It's a wonderfully self-regulating system. The more your child nurses, the more milk you produce. The less your child nurses, the less milk you produce. So, if you're worried about your milk supply, simply nurse more often. Supplementing breast milk with formula short-circuits the whole process. Anything that reduces your baby's hunger or her need to suck will ultimately reduce your milk supply.

♡ Take Care of You: **Have a Drink**

Always have a glass of water, milk, or weak juice by your side. When your baby is drinking, you should be, too.

Baby in Charge

How often you feed will be determined by your baby. Put simply, babies eat when they are hungry and they stop when they are full. The only clock your baby cares about is her own body clock. If she is allowed to follow her own body rhythms throughout her life, she is less likely to become an overweight adult.

At the same time, babies in their first week of life are very sleepy, particularly if labor medications were used during the birth process. If your baby isn't waking on her own every two to three hours during the first week, you'll need to wake her to breastfeed. After the first week of life, your baby will be more wakeful and will begin to tune in to her own body rhythms. Until then, you may have to rouse her to reinforce the feeding pattern.

Suppertime 24/7

At first, it may seem that your newborn is living on your breast. In truth, most newborns spend an average of 187 minutes per day (or three hours) nursing during their first two weeks of life. It seems like a lot because they are on the breast every two to three hours, but each session lasts only fifteen to thirty minutes. Babies also tend to nurse more during growth spurts, which happen around three weeks, six weeks, three months, and six months.

 Smart Mama Tricks: **Name the Act**

Think about what you are going to name the act of breastfeeding because, sooner than you think, your baby will be using that word. Do you really want her repeatedly shouting "tittie" or "boobie" in the grocery store checkout line?

Identifying early hunger cues is an important part of learning to "read" your baby's behavior. Crying is a late hunger cue. If you wait until babies cry, you've waited too long. Anticipate that she will be hungry when she wakes up, or when she displays these cues, night and day:

- Brings her clenched fist to her mouth
- Begins sucking on her fist or fingers
- Roots by turning her head to find your nipple

The "I Have a Life" Guide to Baby's 1st Year

46

- Displays increased activity or movement
- Vocalizes and begins to make noise

♡ Take Care of You: **Involve Your Partner**

Your partner can help you create a nursing nest, bringing you pillows, refilling your drink, offering a paperback book or the telephone (or turning the answering machine on), and if you're really lucky, perhaps even rubbing your feet!

How Do I Know If My Baby's Eating Enough?

Here are some helpful hints to let you know when your baby is full, or not full enough:

- She nurses eight to ten times a day.
- She has six to eight wet diapers a day after the first week. (To understand what "wet diaper" means, pour two ounces of water into a diaper and feel its weight.)
- Her poop resembles Dijon mustard mixed with cottage cheese by the fifth day.
- Your baby seems healthy and alert.
- She gains weight after the first week.
- Your breasts feel full before each feeding and softer afterward.

Common Nursing Dilemmas

From leaky breasts to sore nipples to a biting baby, breastfeeding is not without its occasional challenges. Fortunately, most breastfeeding problems are easily resolved if you catch them early enough.

- **Leaking.** If leaking occurs at all, it most often happens during the first few weeks of breastfeeding; although it can continue throughout the course of your nursing life. To avoid or minimize leakage, use breast pads and/or press against your breasts with your forearm when you begin to feel the tingle that signals a let-down.

- **Sore Nipples.** Sore nipples usually result from improper latch-on or incorrect positioning. Blisters also occur from rubbing against the roof of baby's mouth or along her gums. To treat sore nipples, apply lanolin or express a little breastmilk and dab it on. Ensure that baby always has a good latch, and remember to break suction with your finger.

♡ Take Care of You: **Invest in New Bras**

Avoid common breast problems and discomfort by purchasing and wearing comfortable bras, avoiding underwires or anything that binds or constrains the breasts. Your breasts are probably at least one cup size larger anyway. Give them room to breathe.

- **Plugged Ducts.** A clogged milk duct is fairly obvious—you feel a small lump in your breast, and it can be painful. To treat it, put a warm washcloth over it for five minutes, then massage the lump gently, pushing the milk down toward your nipple. Then start nursing your baby, making sure the baby is positioned so she faces the clogged duct, and continue massaging.

Some common breast ailments that should not be ignored are:

- **Mastitis.** Breast infections are serious. If you have flu-like symptoms, a low fever, red streaks or patches on the breast skin, pain in your breast, or a hard lump in your breast, call your healthcare provider. Mastitis is most often treated with antibiotics. Absolutely do not stop nursing, as that will only make the infection worse.
- **Thrush.** Thrush or candida is a common yeast infection of both moms and babes. Infants with thrush have white patches inside their mouths or an angry rash on their bottoms. Mothers often have sharp, shooting pains in their breasts, and sometimes red, tender nipples or patches of red or white on the breast. See your doctor. Thrush typically responds well to antifungal treatment.
- **Teething and Biting.** Many breastfeeding moms get bitten at least once when the first teeth come in. If you have a biter, use your finger to take the baby off of your breast, say "No" or "Ouch" distinctly and calmly, and hold her off a few seconds before letting her suck again. If baby continues to use you as a human chew toy, offer a safe teething toy instead, to help reinforce its use.

- **Flat or Inverted Nipples.** If your nipples don't protrude when you're aroused—or in a cold breeze—you may have inverted nipples. Truly inverted nipples can prevent successful breastfeeding, but most will respond to treatment—manually rolling your nipples several times a day, wearing a cup inside your bra that presses the areola and encourages the nipple to protrude, or pumping with a heavy-duty pump.

Nursing Strike or Weaning?

A nursing strike is just what it sounds like: a baby's abrupt refusal to breastfeed due to some interfering factor like teething pain, a stuffy nose, or even Mom's new perfume. She'll purse her lips, refuse the breast, and cry—for one feeding or up to several days. Many moms mistake a nursing strike for self-weaning and give up breastfeeding long before their babies are ready. But babies who self-wean usually lose interest gradually over time or are more distractible at the breast. In contrast, most nursing strikes happen suddenly and while babies are still very young.

♡ Take Care of You: **In Case of Interruption**

Some medications are not safe to use while breastfeeding. Ask your pediatrician whether it's safe to continue nursing. If you must temporarily wean due to medication, use a breast pump to maintain your milk production. You'll need to "pump and dump" as often as your baby would nurse.

The solution? If at first you don't succeed, try, try again. Offer the breast when your baby is sleepy. She is less prone to fight it when she's tired. Offer to nurse again as your baby wakes. The quiet-alert state is best. Sometimes simply changing feeding positions or nursing while walking helps.

If your baby still refuses to nurse, express your milk and offer it in an infant feeding cup, a spoon, a syringe, an eyedropper, or a sippy cup.

After twenty-four hours of baby's refusal of the breast, call your doctor or lactation consultant for a checkup to factor out health conditions like thrush or ear infection.

How Long to Breastfeed?

During the first few weeks, you're struggling to figure out how to breastfeed and feeling as if all you do is feed your baby. This is not the time to decide how long you'll breastfeed. Just get going without a stop date in mind. Months will pass. You may add bottles—of breastmilk or formula—to the routine when you go back to work or need some time to yourself.

The current recommendation of the AAP is to breastfeed throughout the first year of your baby's life and then as long as is mutually desirable. Your baby may wean herself before then—or not. You may want to continue breastfeeding into the second year—or not. You may wean to a bottle or find that your baby does just fine with a cup. You may decide to wean because you are pregnant with another child, or choose to continue breastfeeding through your next pregnancy. Once you've made a successful start at breastfeeding, the options for continuing are all yours.

Chapter 5

Diaper Madness

You're expected to know all about taking care of a baby, from washing her hair to cutting her toenails. You might think the most important thing to know is how to give baby a bath. But the bath to diaper-changing ratio suggests that you'll need to know a lot more about diapering than how to bathe her. The average newborn goes through about eight to ten diapers every day. That's about seventy diapers in your first week alone.

Poop Particulars

In your baby's first few days, her poop will look like tar—black, sticky, and hard to remove. This is meconium, a thick, dark green or black paste that fills a baby's intestines in utero and must be eliminated before she can digest normally. If you're lucky, she'll have eliminated most of the meconium in the hospital. If not, you'll be wiping it off at home.

In the transitional stage, your baby's bowel movements will turn yellow-green. If you're breastfeeding, after your milk comes in, your baby's poop will resemble seeded, slightly runny Dijon mustard and smell of buttermilk gone south. If you're formula-feeding, it will be more tan and thicker than peanut butter and smell (putting it kindly) not so sweet.

The most amazing thing about this bodily function is how noisy it can be from such a small person. There you are, holding your precious, dozing baby as relatives coo over how sweet she is, when you hear the sound of a volcano erupting. It's definitely a conversation-stopper, and a clue to run, not walk, to the changing table.

Typically, your baby will dirty several diapers a day. But she may have bowel movements as often as ten times a day. By two to three months, some breastfed babies might only have a bowel movement once a week. Both are normal. The ten-times-a-day baby does not have diarrhea, and the once-a-week-baby is not constipated (unless the poop, when it comes, arrives in pellets). For younger infants, however, especially in their first few weeks of life, not having regular bowel movements can be a sign of a serious problem, and you should check with your provider if you are concerned.

Diaper Wars

Be forewarned: You will need lots of diapers. You may have been perfectly happy to let the nurses deal with diapering at the hospital. Why not? The nurses in the hospital whisked those disposable diapers on and off faster than the eye could see. Once you get home, however, things aren't quite so simple. First, you have to choose sides—are you going to be on Team Cloth or Team Disposable?

There are women who can argue about their diaper choices for hours. One concern is environmental impact (disposables become solid waste that must be disposed of in landfills; cloth diapers use energy and water for laundering, and, if you're using a diaper service, transporting). The other concern is the health of the baby (cloth diapers are more natural and you're likely to change them more often; disposables keep baby drier, but leak synthetic pellets when they get overloaded). And there is a middle road—environmentally sensitive disposable diapers that don't contain chemically synthesized absorbents and/or don't go through chlorine bleaching.

 Smart Mama Tricks: **Aim It Down**

When you're diapering a boy, make sure his penis is pointed down in the center of the diaper. If you accidentally diaper his penis up, or tucked out of a leg edge, you will end up with a wet lap as he directs his spray out of the diaper.

Team Cloth

Cloth diapers are soft and natural and were probably what you were diapered in, since there probably were no disposables when you were a baby. However, cloth diapers have changed significantly since your mother or grandmother used them. Nowadays, there is no need for diaper pins or plastic pants. Modern diapers and diaper covers are mostly made of waterproof, breathable material and have Velcro closures. There are also diaper services that provide you with the diapers, clean them, and return them to you. However, you can still purchase the cloth diapers yourself and do it on your own the old-fashioned way. Whatever way you choose to do it, consider joining a local or online group where advice, information, and support for cloth diapering is shared. And be sure to research the pricing and to find a good deal for quality products.

REASONS TO USE CLOTH DIAPERS

- Cloth diapers have a hundred other uses (including peek-a-boo, burping rag, and eventually dust rag and silver-polisher).
- You'll be more attentive to your baby's needs since you'll have to change her diaper more quickly when she wets.
- Kids may potty train earlier because they can feel the uncomfortable wetness and be more aware of their bodily functions.
- They are less expensive than disposables so you save money (unless you use a higher-end diaper service).
- Fewer chemicals are touching your baby's skin.

Smart Mama Tricks: **Practice Cloth at the Hospital**

If, before the birth of your baby, you already know that you plan to use cloth diapers, bring your cloth-diapering supplies with you to the hospital. Chances are, you can find a nurse to show you the ins and outs of cloth diapering so you can practice before you go home.

Usually a diaper service will give you seventy diapers and a pail. You simply put the dirty diapers in the pail and once a week on a specified day they will take the dirty diapers and give you clean ones.

This option is more expensive than buying and cleaning the diapers yourself, but it saves you the hassle of washing upward of seventy diapers every week.

Team Disposable

Probably one reason disposables are more popular is that putting them on is more intuitive. Open one up with the tapes or Velcro tags underneath your baby, put her bottom in the middle of the diaper, bring the front of the diaper up between her legs, and fasten the tabs at her waist. However, there are even a few tricks to diapering with disposables.

- While your baby still has her umbilical cord, fold the top of the diaper down to turn it into a low-rise bikini before fastening.
- Make sure the leg edges are turned out, not folded back under the elastic. This creates a better seal.
- If your disposables fasten with adhesive tapes, make sure not to get anything on the adhesive—lotions, water, or powder will ruin their stickiness. If your disposables fasten with Velcro tabs, don't pull the tabs too hard, or they might rip off.
- Even though today's disposables are unlikely to leak until they weigh more than your baby, change them once they get a little squishy. Otherwise, the little pellets of super-absorbent gel burst out of the diaper and stick all over your baby's skin.

REASONS TO USE DISPOSABLE DIAPERS

- Disposables are required by most daycare centers and preferred by most caregivers.
- They're less bulky so your baby's clothes will fit better.
- You have less financial commitment up front, and you don't need pins or wraps.
- Used diapers go right out to the trash.
- You'll have fewer changes and less laundry to do.

Diapering A, B, Cs

Make sure you have everything you need within reach before you put your baby on the changing table, countertop, bed, or floor to change her. If your changing table has a strap, slip your hand between your baby's belly and the clip before you try to fasten it to avoid pinching your baby's delicate skin. Use the dirty diaper to do as much preliminary wiping as you can before you bring out the clean cloths or wipes.

Try not to look disgusted; you want your baby to think getting her diaper changed is fun. Plus, you don't want her to think what she has done is a bad thing. Sing, spin a mobile, or hold a toy in your mouth—anything to keep your baby entertained and on her back. Clean the baby's bottom with plain water (using an infant washcloth, cut-up towel, soft paper towel, or cotton balls) for the first month. Save commercial diaper wipes for later as they may irritate your infant's skin.

For a girl, make sure you wipe front to back, using a clean section of washcloth or piece of cotton each time, to prevent spreading bacteria from the poop to the vagina. Although you don't typically need to clean the inside of the lips of the vulva, sometimes it seems as if poop is in every fold, back and front.

For a boy, toss an extra diaper over his penis while you're cleaning him. This reduces your chances of getting squirted in the face.

♡ Take Care of You: Watch Your Back

Make sure your changing surface is tall enough so you don't hurt your back when bending over it.

Remember: Speed counts—the faster you can get your baby diapered and dressed the happier you're both likely to be. Accuracy counts—if the diaper isn't lined up correctly on your baby before you fasten it, it will leak. Treat diaper rash at the first signs—don't let it get out of hand.

When you're done diapering, dump whatever is loose from the dirty diaper into the toilet. This goes for disposable diapers, too. Their biggest environmental hazard may not be the amount of paper in the diapers; a larger concern is the problems caused by leaching bacteria from feces into the ecosystem. By depositing a poop in the toilet, it travels to a treatment plant, rather than to the landfill.

Dry your baby with a clean washcloth or cloth diaper. When you're done, wash your hands well.

Diapering Older Babies

Diapering gets more challenging as your baby gets more control over her body and can kick away your hands, flip over, and, eventually, try to stand up. If she's persistent in wriggling, move the scene of operation to a washable rug on the floor.

 Smart Mama Tricks: **Special Diaper-Time Toys**

To keep things simple (and to keep an older baby's roving hands away from a soiled area), use distraction as much as possible. Have a special toy she gets to hold only at diaper time (make sure it's light in case she drops it on herself), sing special songs, make faces.

You may have to swing a leg over her torso to gently pin her to the floor during some of the wrigglier stages. And once your baby learns to stand up, you may have to learn to change her diaper while she's vertical.

Diaper Rash

Diaper rash can be as mild as a little redness or as severe as bleeding sores. Some babies seem to get it all the time; others hardly ever. Peak diaper-rash times are when babies start to eat solid foods, when they sleep through the night in a dirty diaper, and when they are taking antibiotics. The best way to treat it is to prevent it.

Change diapers frequently (immediately if they're messy). Expose your baby's bottom to air and light as often as you can. When your baby's an infant, this is pretty easy. In a warm room, put her belly down on a disposable absorbent pad (the kind you sat on in the hospital) or use a waterproof crib pad with a cloth diaper on top of it. Once your baby is mobile, it is less likely she'll stay put. If it's summer, let her run around bare-bottomed outside (using common sun-sense, of course). If it's winter, you might consider warming up your bathroom and giving her a little extra naked time after her bath.

What you shouldn't have to do to prevent diaper rash is slather on ointment with every single diaper change.

 ## Smart Mama Tricks: No "Wipes" for Rashes

If your baby has graduated to wipes, you should go back to using plain warm water to clean your baby's bottom while she's rashy. Diaper wipes may make the rash worse.

If you notice a little redness—the beginnings of diaper rash—begin treating it immediately. Don't just hope it will go away on it's own; it's likely to get worse, becoming a lot more uncomfortable for your baby and a lot harder for you to treat. If the rash doesn't go away, especially if it is bright red and surrounded by small red bumps, then it may be a yeast infection. Ask your pediatrician to prescribe an antifungal ointment.

Chapter 6

Body and Soul

In the weeks that follow the birth of your baby, the initially constant flow of blood from your vagina will slow to a trickle and then stop. Your breasts will adjust to nursing—or not nursing—and will cease to feel like foreign objects attached to your body. You may not be getting much sleep, but you'll get used to surviving on whatever sleep you do get. And you'll soon be out of those first- or second-trimester maternity clothes and back into something more stylish.

Lost Your Mind?

Teary, overwhelmed, and strange is typical in the postpartum weeks—and sometimes months. You could have dramatic mood swings. You may cry for no reason at all and might feel unable to cope with situations you would usually handle just fine. You may explode in anger when those around you least expect it.

This is normal. It's natural to have an emotional reaction to a major life change—and a new baby is a major life change. You're stressed by the demands placed on you as a new mother, and daunted by the responsibility that is suddenly, literally, in your lap. Of course you're exhausted when your sleep is constantly interrupted. You're also reacting physically and emotionally to the dramatic postpartum change in your hormone levels.

Some scientists say it's the same type of reaction as premenstrual syndrome (PMS). You can't avoid this hormone drop. It's how your body returns to normal.

It's Temporary

There's not much you can do about hormone fluctuations except hang on for the ride. However, there are a few handy tips that can help you deal with the mood swings and physical exhaustion, mainly eating well, sleeping when you can, drinking lots of liquids, and asking for help from family or friends. It will be short-lived. For most new mothers, the hardest part is the first few days. If you can manage to laugh at some of the ridiculous things you think and feel during those first few days, the rest will be a breeze.

♡ Take Care of You: "Me" Time

Hand the baby off to your partner after dinner and soak in the bathtub—for hours. Or meet a friend and see a movie. Try to have a regularly scheduled time where your partner takes the baby and you take some much needed "me" time.

For some women, the hormonal changes may be too extreme to handle without a doctor's help and/or medication. If you fit into that category, you're not a wimp; you're just chemically out of whack.

Baby Blues or Postpartum Depression?

During the first weeks after birth, many women experience minor depressive episodes lasting anywhere from a few hours to a few weeks. These are usually bouts of the baby blues.

Postpartum depression, or PPD, also surfaces within the first weeks after childbirth but is more severe than the baby blues. It lasts longer and feels more intense. Unlike the baby blues, which merely take time to pass, PPD usually requires medical treatment.

How can you tell if you need more help than your best friend, mother, or babysitter can give you? Signs you may need medical help include:

- You can't sleep at night, even when the baby does
- Lack of appetite
- Loss of interest in activities you usually enjoy
- Lack of enthusiasm for anything
- Difficulty making decisions
- Constant anxiety about your baby
- General anxiety
- Recurrent, strong feelings of anger
- Recurrent crying, tearfulness
- Feelings of hopelessness
- Feelings of inadequacy
- Disaster fantasies
- Shaking
- Compulsive behaviors

- Panic attacks (shortness of breath, dizziness)
- Sleeping too little or too much
- Suicidal thoughts*
- Thoughts about harming the baby*

    If you are having suicidal thoughts or thoughts about harming your baby, tell your doctor or a trusted friend immediately.

If you are experiencing an increasing number of these symptoms, and they intensify with time, make sure you get all the help you need. Tell the people in your life who are most likely to take action to get you some relief. Include at least one relative or close friend and one health care provider, and enlist support sooner than later. Seeking help when you need it is a sign of strength, not of weakness.

Stress-Stopping Toolbox

Your physical and mental health is critical to successful parenting. With that in mind, remember to do at least a few of the following every day:

Breathe deeply. Lie on your bed and take deep abdominal cleansing breaths. Focus on your breathing. Try yoga.

Eat right and eat light. High-protein foods like nuts, seeds, and beans will increase your energy level. So will iron-rich foods like eggs, red meat, fish, poultry, whole grain cereals and breads, dried fruits, and legumes. Drink a glass of orange juice with these. Vitamin C helps your body absorb iron more efficiently.

Exercise. Your body releases endorphins after several minutes of exercise. Endorphins are your body's natural painkillers; they make you feel good about yourself and give you a natural high. Once you have your six-week clearance from your doctor, put your newborn in a sling or stroller and start walking.

Laugh! Rent a funny movie, read a humorous book, visit a joke Web site, or talk to a friend who makes you giggle. Laughter is indeed the best medicine.

Get a massage. A good massage reduces the stress hormone known as cortisol. It also boosts your immune system, alleviates stress, helps you relax, and induces sleep. And it feels so good.

Prioritize. Is it more important to take care of yourself or your laundry? This is a busy time for you. Think about what really matters most. Now that you are a family, work may have to wait.

Sleep. There is no better way to reenergize than to take catnaps whenever possible. Sleep when baby sleeps. Or lie down together and breastfeed. As a new parent, you probably won't have any trouble falling asleep, but if you do, try eating healthy bedtime snacks that induce sleep, like a slice of turkey on a bagel with a glass of warm milk.

Take vitamins. Your prenatal vitamins contain minerals like magnesium, folic acid, and zinc. Those, coupled with B and C vitamins, will help maintain your body's energy. Vitamins alone can't accomplish what a healthy, balanced diet can, so use these in conjunction with nutritious foods.

Talk. Your frustrations are real. Call a friend, a parent, or a crisis line, if needed. Join a moms' group. Develop new support systems with people who have previous experience in parenting. Surround yourself with positive people.

Step outside. Fresh air can work wonders for a distressed spirit.

Postpartum Elation

This is one postpartum emotion that rarely makes the news. Postpartum elation can include the sheer joy of being a new mother, the thrill of surviving labor and delivery, and the pride you feel when you look at your new baby. When you feel postpartum elation, you won't be able to stop talking about how happy you are. You'll be sharing your birth story with everyone in the hospital, in the supermarket, on the bus. No, it's not all pain and misery.

I Want My Body Back!

Although technically you don't need your old body back in order to have a life, how you feel about your body has a direct impact on your self-esteem. If you're not loving yourself, that can lead to all kinds of problems, the least of which means you may not want to get out and about as often.

This may be addressed in two ways: One, try to come to terms with the beautiful body you have now, the one that carried your child and likely nourishes him as well. Two, work a healthy diet and an exercise routine into this new life of yours, so you can gradually get back into shape. Rest assured that although you might not get your old body back, you can get a body you like.

♡ Take Care of You: **Water, Water Everywhere**

Water is the recommended beverage. Juice and soft drinks are too sugary and don't replace your body's fluids as well as water does. A glass or two of fruit juice per day may be a healthy addition to your diet, but drinking juice instead of water can lead to unwanted weight gain.

Postpartum Body Blues

One of the biggest surprises to hit new moms right after birth is their belly. The baby doesn't live there anymore, but why isn't your tummy back to normal? Why does it look like a saggy, squishy sack attached to your midsection? Most new moms will need to live in their first- or second-trimester maternity clothes for a while after birth. Rest assured that your midsection will shrink down during this postpartum period—to what degree varies from woman to woman.

Be careful not to lose more than one to one-and-a-half pounds per week. More rapid weight loss is not safe for you or your baby, and the more gradually you can lose weight, the better off you will both be. Remember, it took nine months to put on the excess weight your body needed during pregnancy and it basically takes at least that amount of time for your body to return to normal.

But at the same time, remember that some things will never go back to the way they were. Your uterus will always be a little larger than before, the opening of the cervix wider, and your pelvic muscles and ligaments looser. Your waist and hips might not return all the way to pre-pregnancy size, and many women's feet remain larger—you may have to throw out a lot of shoes. Some women return to their pre-pregnancy weight, or even below that, but find that things are, well, redistributed. Your skin might be stretched out around your abdomen, your breasts may remain larger or they may become smaller than pre-pregnancy after you wean your child. If your baby had a favorite breast and nursed more on one side, you may find yourself permanently lopsided.

♡ Take Care of You: Postpartum Birth Control

Be sure to discuss birth control with your provider. Even if you haven't yet gotten your period, you can still get pregnant. Remember, you can be fertile before your first period. The safest choices when you're breastfeeding are nonchemical, such as condoms, diaphragms, and cervical caps.

If you're breastfeeding, you probably won't get your period back for several months. Although some women who breastfeed exclusively get their periods back much sooner and some not until their baby weans.

Hair Today, Gone Tomorrow

You're standing in the shower—shampoo, rinse, repeat—and suddenly clumps of hair come off in your hands. This, too, is normal. For a while when you were pregnant, your hair was thicker than ever due to changes in the shedding cycle. The bad news is that this too will pass, and you'll lose the normal amount of hair you would have had you not been pregnant—all at once.

Sometimes your hair will grow back in a little fringe around your hairline, coming in like baby hair. The time it takes for your hair to look "normal" again depends on your hair's growth cycle, which can vary dramatically from woman to woman. Get a good haircut or some nice scarves and have faith; it will grow back.

Occupational Hazards

Just like with any vocation, motherhood comes with its fair share of on-the-job injuries. Learn how to avoid these mom-specific concerns.

Baby Wrist

Given all the holding, cuddling, and cradling that babies require, it's no surprise that some mothers suffer from a condition sometimes called baby wrist. This is a repetitive stress injury, characterized by pain or tingling in the wrist that can cause long-term damage if not treated. A variation is pain around the thumb or fingers, which doctors now associate with lifting and carrying the baby. The pain often increases at night, when the accumulation of fluid increases the pressure on the nerves.

♡ Take Care of You: **Prevent "Baby Wrist"**

If you are feeling pain from holding your baby, consider carrying him in a sling or front pack more often to take the load off of your wrists. For a larger baby, try a backpack or try a hip-carrying position in a sling.

You can head off the condition by stretching your wrists regularly and lifting light hand weights. Make sure you keep your wrists in a "neutral" position (straight, but relaxed), when holding your baby, whether you're carrying him, holding his head while nursing, or pushing a stroller.

My Aching Back

While you were pregnant, you began to carry yourself differently to balance your growing stomach. Continuing this new posture can strain your back, as can nursing (remember to use a nursing stool and bring your baby to your breast, rather than leaning over your baby) and the constant lifting and carrying a new baby needs.

To minimize the stress on your back, rediscover your correct posture. Stand in front of a mirror, naked, and close your eyes. Rock from side to side, shrug your shoulders, take a slow, deep breath, and exhale. Then, without opening your eyes, try to find a centered position. Open your eyes and look in the mirror. To adjust your alignment, put your feet just under your hips, then tip your pelvis forward and back until you find its center. Tuck in your bottom, and straighten your shoulders. You may need to do this a few times a day until you get used to your new center.

Become aware of how you hold and handle your baby. When you bend down to pick her up, bend your knees, support her close to your chest, and use your leg muscles to lift—don't lean over. The same goes for the car seat. Climb into the car as far as possible and sit if you can. Then lift your baby up against you before squirming backward out of the car.

Once your baby is too big for the sink or baby tub (which you can place on a counter), think about taking baths with your baby instead of leaning over the tub. When you are on the floor changing a diaper or playing, squat or sit cross-legged to reduce awkward leaning. Try to carry your baby in the center of your body as much as possible, rather than on one hip. Or, if you carry your baby on your hip, switch sides often (the same goes for carrying your baby in a sling).

Exercise

If you hadn't started exercising before pregnancy, it's not too late to start. There are a lot of good reasons to exercise—to stay healthy, to boost your mood, and to fit into your pre-pregnancy clothes again. It's time to get back in touch with your body. To put on, for an hour anyway, clothes you can't nurse in, look in the mirror, and recognize that the leg you are lifting is actually yours. Just check first with your provider to make sure you're ready to begin.

Keep up the Kegels!

Immediately after the birth (or as soon as you have any feeling down in your pelvis) start Kegeling again. Your vagina was stretched by childbirth, and you might worry your vagina will never regain its pre-delivery size. You might wonder whether your partner will find sex less satisfying than before. However, the vagina is a truly remarkable organ. It can expand to accommodate a baby's head and then shrink back to its normal size in just a few days. If you want to accelerate this process along, do your Kegels!

1. Tense up your vaginal and anal muscles as if you were trying to control the flow of urine
2. Hold the tension for three to five seconds
3. Relax and repeat three to five times.

Do these at least a few times a day—and do them for the rest of your life.

Workout Dos and Don'ts

Once your doctor gives the okay, you can also start easy exercises for your lower back and abdomen, though you won't have much success even feeling where your abdominal muscles are for a week or two. Make sure, however, that you don't do any exercises that require you to be upside down until all bleeding stops (no shoulder stands, for example, if you're doing yoga), because blood flowing back into the still-open cervix can cause infection. Nurse just before you exercise; you'll be more comfortable.

Breastfeeding, which uses about 500 to 1,000 calories a day, should help you lose weight, but plan on dropping the pounds slowly. If you're thinking about dieting yourself back into shape and you're significantly overweight, do so only if you mean dieting by controlling your eating. Focus on eating reasonable portions of healthy foods at regular meals. If "dieting" to you means a restrictive fad or starvation diet (living on protein shakes or grapefruit), don't—you'll threaten your baby's health as well as your own.

Yoga Baby

Postpartum yoga classes are a fabulous way to get exercise with your baby, as well as to meet other new moms. Check your local yoga studios and parenting circles in your community to find them. Some offer mom/infant classes only until baby reaches the crawling stage; others offer separate classes for pre-crawlers and crawlers.

While your infant lies contentedly on a blanket beside you, you entertain him with your gentle and invigorating yoga poses—or not. You'll notice that during the class, several mothers may be nursing, changing diapers, or comforting crying babies. And you yourself may be doing any number of these activities on any given day. One class, you may get a full forty-five minutes of actual yoga in. Another day, you might get ten minutes and nurse your baby the rest of the time. Continue to attend the yoga class regularly anyway. The stretching, strengthening, and supportive camaraderie of the other moms are some of the best things you can do for yourself.

Take a Hike

Most experienced moms will tell you: Walking is key. It's something you can do with your baby that your baby usually enjoys, too. It gets you both out in the fresh air (or if the weather is bad, out to the local mall), it's safe, and it's cardiovascular. By yourself, with a friend, or with an organized group, it's the easiest way to burn calories and rebuild your strength. The added endorphin boost feels great, too.

Stroller Baby

If you like group activities and find yourself more motivated in a class situation, these workouts may be just the thing. You get together with anywhere from a few to more than a dozen other moms or dads with babies in strollers and power-walk a course, stopping at various points along the way for body toning exercises. Stroller Strides is one of the best-known nationwide programs. Their trained fitness instructors (who are moms, too) provide a full-body workout and, depending on the group, sometimes offer playgroup activities for the youngsters and other social activities as well. For more information, visit *www.strollerstrides.com*.

An Exercise Opportunist

With all of the new responsibilities of parenthood, clearing your schedule at a certain time every day or two for exercise isn't always practical. It's easy to get so busy that you forget to take care of yourself. Everyone else's needs seem to come first. Your baby needs to be fed, changed, and held. Your toddler needs attention, stimulation, and socialization. In those busy first months, you've got to become an exercise opportunist.

♡ Take Care of You: **Early Morning Workout**

Try getting up half an hour before your baby's usual wake-up time and working out. You'll find that you're energized, not exhausted.

Make exercise part of your ordinary activities. Three ten-minute blocks of time are as effective as 30 minutes in a row. Shorter stretches are easier to get through and easier to schedule. Even little activities that seem like they wouldn't make much of a difference add up quickly over the course of a few months.

- Do five or ten situps in the morning when you first get up from bed. Add an extra situp every few days.
- Use the stairs instead of the escalator.
- Park at the far end of the parking lot (but always be safe!).
- Choose to stand instead of sit.
- Flex your muscles and hold them tight for a moment while you sit in traffic.
- Run in place.
- Tighten Kegel muscles just about anywhere.
- Tackle the housework. Laundry, dishes, taking out the garbage, washing windows, and vacuuming the floor are productive workouts.

- Do the yard work. Let your partner watch the baby while you weed, mow, or shovel.

After you and your baby have negotiated a sleep schedule, you can start to enjoy more traditional workouts a few times per week. It's hard for new parents to imagine having the time for a formal workout, but remember that exercise only seems like it takes time. It really saves time.

Exercise sharpens both your mind and body, helping you cut through your tasks more quickly with less effort. The little bit of time you spend on exercise will pay you back many times over with increased efficiency.

Consistency Is Key

Even if you think you have no time to exercise, even if you used to work out 90 minutes a day four days a week before you had a baby, every little bit you do now counts. If you can only do your postpartum yoga DVD once a week during baby's 30-minute catnap, do it. Every week. This seemingly insignificant bit of exercise will add up over time. You will find the workout getting easier, and yourself getting stronger. You don't need large blocks of time to exercise. Fact is, you don't have large blocks of time anymore. Do the small-scale short workouts, but do them regularly. It will make all the difference.

Chapter 7

To Sleep or Not to Sleep

Whats usually the most pressing issue for a new parent? Sleep. How to get baby to "sleep through the night," how to get enough sleep yourself, and how to survive when you're sleep-deprived. It can be hard to have a life, even a new and exciting one, when you're sleepwalking through it like a zombie. The fact is, your sleep cycle will be affected. Just how much remains to be seen. In truth, there are no easy answers or miracle cures to the baby/sleep dilemma. It's often just a matter of the luck of the draw.

Sleepyhead

Your baby will sleep a lot his first year. Not precisely when you want him to, of course, but he'll sleep about sixteen or seventeen hours total per day during his first month (give or take a few hours), and gradually decrease to about fourteen hours by his first birthday. And no, not all of that sleep time will be at night. Early on, instead of long stretches of sleep, your newborn will likely have fairly regular cycles of eating, sleeping, and waking each day. Although there might be one longer stretch of four or five hours, most of these cycles will be just two or three hours.

The first six weeks are frequently the toughest for the parents, as it's not until around the age of six weeks that your baby starts differentiating day from night, sleeping longer during the nighttime while remaining awake for longer stretches during the day.

Over the next three or four months, your baby's sleep patterns should become more organized. He will still be sleeping a lot, but there will be more sleep at night, longer periods of wakefulness during the day, and more regular nap times. Don't be alarmed if these transitions take place earlier or later in your baby. Such variations are normal.

♡ Take Care of You: It's Not Forever

Remember that infancy is temporary and fleeting. Your baby will grow older and stronger and will sleep through the night. Rest assured that the day will eventually arrive, and take comfort in realizing that every new dawn brings you one day closer to that milestone.

Just as your baby's sleep patterns change over this first year, sleep advice also changes. Realize that much of the usual advice for older children—letting them fall asleep on their own, not letting them fall asleep while feeding, and perhaps even letting them cry it out—does not apply to your newborn or young baby. Your newborn probably will fall asleep breast-feeding or drinking a bottle or may need to be rocked to sleep. Helping your child get to sleep in these first few months doesn't mean that you are creating problems for later.

All Night Long

Fact: Infants need to eat at night as well as during the day. Your newborn will likely continue to feed every two to three hours (or more often) at night, just as he does during the day. If you're lucky, he might go for one long stretch of four to five hours at night without nursing or taking a bottle, but in general, count on waking up for several nighttime feedings, at least in the early days.

Sleeping through the night is really only possible when your baby is neurologically ready. It cannot be forced by feeding your baby cereal, letting your baby cry, or any other rumored "cure." Approach any "surefire methods" to make your baby sleep through the night with skepticism.

♡ Take Care of You: Midnight Anger Amnesty

Make a deal with Daddy that heated comments exchanged under duress in the middle of the night (e.g., while holding a screaming baby or changing the second blowout diaper since midnight) will not be taken seriously. You're both tired and need to give each other a break.

Avoid the Comparison Trap

Adults have different sleep patterns; the same is true among babies. Though certain patterns are average, a deviation from that pattern is usually quite normal. So when your cousin's best friend's wife's four-month-old sleeps more, or less, or simply at different hours than your child, don't worry about it. We're all different—babies, too.

Breathing Room

Choosing sleeping arrangements and bedtimes is challenging. The more sleep you lose, the harder it is to think rationally on this topic. Your decision depends on your lifestyle, your beliefs, your baby.

Smart Mama Tricks: **Back to Sleep**

Regardless of where baby sleeps, always place baby to sleep on his back, according to American Academy of Pediatrics recommendations. Studies have shown that back sleeping is related to a lower incidence of Sudden Infant Death Syndrome (SIDS).

Your baby's bedtime will most likely change as he gets older. In the beginning, try to keep the same hours as your baby. For example, if your baby tends to launch into his one five-hour stretch of sleep a night at 7:00 P.M., go to bed at the same time so you can get a chunk of sleep, as well. (Even if you can't go to bed at this hour, at least lie down and take a nap.) You may miss your favorite TV shows or some time alone with your partner, but understand that this is temporary and absolutely necessary if you want to function well. You'll be glad you crashed early when your baby pops awake at 4:00 A.M., ready to begin his day.

The Family Bed

Co-sleeping, or having your baby sleep in bed with you, is the natural way to parent at night. This is the way babies have slept throughout most of history and still do in many parts of the world. This sleeping arrangement enables parents to respond quickly to the child's needs. Many parents enjoy the comfort and security of having baby right there with them.

Co-sleeping, also called sleep sharing or the family bed, must be executed using common sense and following strict safety guidelines. It can be beneficial for you as well as your baby and will not cause your baby to become dependent on you to sleep. Your child will eventually leave your bed when you are both ready.

Upside

What are the advantages of having your baby in your bed? To begin with, babies are soothed by the touch of their parents at any time, day or night, awake or asleep. If baby wakes during the night with the sniffles, you'll wake up and hear him quickly. If the baby spits up, you'll know that, too. You won't unknowingly leave him lying all night in a crib that he's spit up into, with regurgitated milk that's now going sour.

If the room is too warm or too cold, you'll be aware of it, since you're in the same room and the same bed as baby is. If your baby wakes from a bad dream, you are right there beside him. He may not scream or cry or even whimper. Feeling, smelling, or seeing (if you use a night-light) the familiar forms of his parents beside him, he will very possibly feel secure enough to close his eyes and work his way back to sleep, without the terror he might have felt otherwise and without waking you up.

Smart Mama Tricks: Background Noise

Some babies, like some parents, are light sleepers. If this is your child and you don't want to live in a hush of silence at naptime every day, try plugging in an air filter or turning on the clothes dryer near the baby's room or playing a restful song on repeat, to create noise that will mask the other sounds in the house and ensure a peaceful, uninterrupted sleep.

More seriously, if your baby starts to choke, you'll hear him right away and be able to help him. Should he stop breathing, be it from sleep apnea, from SIDS, or from some other cause, you may realize it, wake up with a start, and be able to take measures to try to get him breathing again right away.

Perhaps the greatest beneficiaries of a family bed sleeping arrangement are the nursing baby and his mom. When your infant wakes up beside you during the night and is hungry or just wants to suckle a little for the relaxation he needs to help himself back to sleep, he can latch on to a nipple and begin to feed. Some mothers under these circumstances don't even wake up or awaken just barely, take note of the fact that the baby is feeding, and go back to sleep. It's so much less disturbing to your sleep than having to get up, retrieve the baby from the crib (even if his crib is in your room), sit down somewhere (whether it's your bed or a chair or the living room sofa) to hold the baby and nurse him, then get up, return him to his crib, and return to your bed, by which time you're fully wide-awake and may lie in bed quite a while before you can get back to sleep.

If you're feeding your baby infant formula, you can still have some of the ease of breastfeeding if you co-sleep. You can keep the formula by the side of the bed and simply reach for it when he wakes to feed.

♡ Take Care of You: **Watch Your Back**

When nursing in the side-lying position in bed, be sure to move baby to the breast, not the other way around. If you are arching your back, you are moving your breast to your baby and you could wake with a sore back.

Should your co-sleeping baby sleep between the two of you or on the outside of one of you? Clearly the baby sleeping between you has little chance of rolling out of bed during the night—but he has two parents who need to be wary of rolling over onto him. If he sleeps between you and the edge, only you need to sleep aware of the hazard, and moms in general are much more sensitive to their babies during the night. In most cases, baby is safer co-sleeping on a mattress on the floor between mom and the edge of the mattress. If you keep your bed elevated, install a mesh bed rail and place baby between mom and the rail. (Ensure there are no gaps between the bed rail and the mattress—if there are, fill them in firmly and completely with rolled up towels or blankets.)

Downside

You may find several disadvantages to having your baby in your bed. When he wakes up during the night, resettles, and goes back to sleep, the slight sounds he makes may wake you up, even though he doesn't need attention. On the other hand, when you are getting ready for bed and when you get up in the morning, the sounds you make, from squeaking bedsprings as you settle down to the ringing of your alarm clock in the morning to the conversations you have with your partner, may all awaken your baby. If he's a very light sleeper, he might wake up every time one of you rolls over and resettles. If he's that light a sleeper, he might do better in his own crib and not in a family bed.

 Smart Mama Tricks: **Bedside Bassinet**

If you want your newborn close by for security and those frequent early feedings, have limited bedroom space, but don't want him in your bed, try using a bassinet for the first several weeks. It takes up much less room than a crib, is much cozier for a newborn, and you can transfer baby to a crib later on, once he outgrows the bassinet.

If your baby wakes up before you do in the morning and he's alone in his own room, he may play happily in his crib for a little while or just lie there contentedly. But if he sees you lying within his view, even though you're still asleep, he's more likely to start to fuss and demand attention.

If the baby is used to having you next to him when he sleeps, he's likely to be unable to fall asleep unless at least one of you is lying beside him. You may need to stretch out on the bed next to your baby every night and stay there at least until he is in his first deep sleep—which is likely to be half an hour for a baby under six months old, though within ten minutes or so for a baby older than that, if you're lucky. Be aware that this may go on for a few years.

♡ Take Care of You: **Nurse to Sleep with Books on Tape**

If your baby takes a long time to nurse down to sleep at night or for his nap, and you feel like you're spending agonizing, impatient minutes lying beside him in the dark, try listening to recorded books on an iPod, MP3, or portable CD player. Time will fly by and you will feel like you got some valuable "me" time, as well.

If your baby wets the bed, it's your bed, and the sheets you have to change are much larger and more cumbersome than changing a crib sheet, and three people's sleep (or more, if you have another child sleeping in with you) will be disturbed so you can change the sheets.

Last, but certainly not least, you and/or your spouse may feel more inhibited about lovemaking when your baby is in the same room.

The Family Bed Safety Debate

Co-sleeping has become the subject of much controversy in the United States. The strong "attachment parenting" childrearing movement has recently spawned a resurgence in this type of sleep arrangement. Although advocates praise the benefits of a family bed, other people question how safe it is and say that it may increase the risk of SIDS. While the American Academy of Pediatrics (AAP) and the Consumer Product Safety Commission (CPSC) are against co-sleeping, there are many other experts who highly recommend the practice. Most notable of these is the respected pediatrician and bestselling author, Dr. William Sears.

If you choose to co-sleep, you're obligated to make the experience as safe for your baby as possible. The CPSC has said of infant mortalities associated with adult beds that, "One of the most tragic aspects of these deaths is that they are largely preventable."

Bed-Sharing Safety Tips

The same safety measures and standards that apply to cribs should apply to your bed.

- Keep the bed away from walls and other furniture (to eliminate the danger of baby getting trapped between the bed and the wall, or the bed and other objects).
- Use an ultrafirm mattress, purchasing a new one if necessary.
- Keep all pillows and other soft bedding items away from baby. (Consider eliminating these items entirely from the bed until baby is at least two years old.)

- Keep the room warm enough that you need only a light blanket. (No heavy blankets, quilts, down comforters, or anything that might smother your baby if he gets down underneath the covers.)
- Get the biggest bed you can (a king or California king is best). If you must use a queen bed, consider putting a twin mattress adjacent to your mattress, so Dad has extra room to sleep (make sure your baby does not sleep where he could roll into the gap between the mattresses).
- If possible, eliminate headboards and footboards to avoid entrapment. (If this is not possible, follow the same rule regarding the spacing of these items as you would the spacing of crib slats.)
- If possible, place your mattress directly on the floor, to avoid long falls.
- Keep the room smoke-free.
- Do not leave baby unattended in bed with a sibling.
- Don't go to bed after drinking alcohol or taking medication.
- Do not co-sleep if you are obese.
- Never co-sleep on a waterbed.

Bed-Sharing with Siblings

Always have an adult positioned between a baby and an older sibling if you all share a bed. Though the older sibling will surely be much smaller and weigh much less than either you or your partner, he will also be much less aware, and so the baby is at greater risk from him rolling over on him than he is from either you or your partner doing so.

Sidecars and Snuggle Nests

If you want baby close by, but not actually in your bed, try one of the sidecar-style co-sleepers. A co-sleeper attaches to the side of your bed as an extension to the bed itself. It resembles a three-sided crib, with the open side adjacent to the bed and the mattress at the same height as the bed mattress. It gives the infant his own space, yet he lies within arms reach. You'll have to pick up the baby and bring him close to breastfeed, but you won't have to get out of bed to do it. Most sidecar co-sleeper manufacturers recommend their use only until baby begins to move around—read the instructions and warnings carefully. Always ensure that there are no gaps between the co-sleeper and your bed where the baby could get trapped.

Infant bed inserts, such as the Snuggle Nest, are protective inserts that are placed in the bed to keep baby in one spot and to help to prevent Mom or Dad from rolling over on baby. If you are concerned about rollover, you might consider one of these. However, if Dad is a heavy sleeper or seems to sleep unaware of your infant, this insert won't be enough to protect your baby—don't gain a false sense of security from the insert alone.

Behind Bars: The Crib

Putting your baby in a crib has its own benefits. You may find that you sleep better with more room and without a squirming, kicking bundle beside you. If you can't sleep for fear of squishing the baby or have a panic attack every time he makes a noise, a crib would work better for you. You may also prefer to keep your bed a private place for you and your partner.

Of course, choose a crib that meets the most current safety standards to prevent injury to your baby, particularly if you purchase a "used" crib or inherit a "hand-me-down" one. Older cribs may pose problems, such as slats spaced too far apart, causing an entrapment hazard; corner posts, knobs, or details that can catch on baby's clothing or come loose and be swallowed; or lead-based paint or other toxic materials. If you obtain an older crib, buy a firm new crib mattress that fits snugly. (You should not be able to fit more than two fingers between the mattress and the sides of the crib.)

 Smart Mama Tricks: **Make a Break for It**

You'll know when your baby moves from REM sleep to non-REM sleep. His eyes will stop moving, his body parts will stop moving and twitching, and at that point you should be able to escape without his waking up and realizing you've decamped for the kitchen or the living room.

Where do you put the crib? Some parents opt to place it in their own bedroom, others in the baby's bedroom. This, again, is a matter of personal choice, whether you are more comfortable being close by to hear and see your baby during the night and to make nighttime feeding sojourns that much easier, or whether having the crib in the same room impedes a bit too much on your personal space and needs. Note that at the time of this writing, the AAP recommends that infants sleep in the same room as their parents. When baby is not sleeping in your bed or even in your room, you still need to be physically responsive to him at any time of night. Make sure he is close enough so you can hear any sounds of distress.

 Smart Mama Tricks: **Layer the Sheets**

Consider placing two or more sets of tight-fitting fitted sheets and waterproof pads in your bassinet or crib. If baby wets the sheets, you need only remove top fitted sheet and top waterproof pad and you're good to go. Only do this if all of the layers still fit snugly and won't come loose.

Sleeping Through the Night

For most parents, having a baby who sleeps well all night long is their ultimate goal. After all, if your baby is sleeping well, then you're probably sleeping well, too. So when will your baby start sleeping through the night? That really depends on what you mean by "sleeping through the night." Some parents think that's a good ten- or eleven-hour stretch without waking up. Other parents are happy with six or eight hours and consider that to be sleeping through the night, because that means that they are getting a nice long stretch of uninterrupted sleep. Many health care professionals define "sleeping through the night" as only five hours.

Whatever your definition, understand that "sleeping through the night" is a bit of a misnomer. We all, adults and babies alike, wake up, however briefly, at least several times during the night. If we get back to sleep quickly, when we wake up in the morning, we don't remember having awakened during the night at all. Babies, too, awaken during the night a few times. They all do. But some can roll over and go back to sleep on their own. Other babies, once they wake up, cannot get themselves back to sleep and cry out.

The trick with your older baby isn't to get him to literally sleep through the night, but rather to help him learn to go back to sleep on his own when he wakes up. Were you paying attention? If you are sleep-deprived, you might have missed that. To repeat: At some point, your older baby needs to be able to go back to sleep on his own when he wakes up. Children reach this milestone at different ages, and there are different schools of thought about helping baby achieve this goal.

♡ Take Care of You: Weekend Sleep-Ins

On Saturday and/or Sunday mornings, have your partner or another trusted adult take baby out of the house for a few hours as soon as the child wakes up. Stay in bed. Close your eyes. Sleeeeeeep.

Parenting to Sleep

Let's start with helping your infant down to sleep in the first place. Dr. Sears suggests nursing or rocking the baby into a sound sleep before putting him down, either in a crib or in your bed. Whenever the baby wakes up, you should get to the baby quickly, he says, since you'll probably have an easier time getting the baby back to sleep if he doesn't scream himself into hysteria first. Here's where having the baby in bed with you is an advantage—you can often soothe or even breastfeed your baby without fully coming awake yourself. Don't worry about building a bad habit in a baby who is under three months old. If it works for tonight, it's good enough.

♡ Take Care of You: **Don't Watch the Clock**

Don't lie in bed, processing what time it is, how many hours you've been awake, how long the baby just nursed, how many times he's already nursed tonight, how many more hours to go until morning— it's non-productive and, worse, will take you that much further from the sleep you need. As hard as it is, face that clock away from you, close your eyes, and don't do the math.

Other experts advise putting baby down when he is almost, but not quite, asleep. The idea behind this theory is that baby learns to go to sleep the rest of the way by himself, and that you can gradually build on this behavior. Eventually, you will be able to put him down when he is tired, but still awake, and allow him to fall asleep on his own. If this works for you, meaning baby doesn't scream as soon as you put him down, count yourself one of the lucky ones. The rest of you will be nursing or rocking or bottle-feeding your infant all the way into a deep sleep.

Time for Bed

It often helps when you put baby to sleep at around the same time every night, preferably following a predictable pre-bedtime ritual. Babies, just like us, get tired and reach a point when they're "ready" for sleep. It's much easier to get your baby to sleep when he's ready than to put him in for the night or for a nap when you want him to sleep but he's feeling wide awake.

Whenever possible, try to stick to baby's own natural sleep pattern. If he's naturally ready to go to sleep at 6:00 P.M., don't plan his feeding time for 6:00 P.M. and bedtime for 7:00 P.M. By the same token, if he's a child who's ready for bed at 7:00 P.M., don't try to put him to bed at 6:00 P.M.

Be wary of becoming a slave to a schedule—particularly if it's a schedule randomly set by you and particularly if you have a younger baby. Infants sleep when they are tired; let them sleep when they want to sleep.

 Smart Mama Tricks: **Napping in the Family Bed**

Even if you all sleep in a family bed, consider having baby take his naps in a crib to ensure he does not wake up and roll into trouble while you are out of the room. If you don't have a crib or other safer nap space, invest in a baby video monitor, so you can see that he remains safely in bed at all times.

If you must change baby's sleep pattern, for example, baby is going to sleep at 5:30 P.M. and getting up at 5:30 A.M. and you are desperate for him to get up later, try to make changes in 10-minute increments. The first day, put him to sleep at 5:40 P.M., then 5:50 P.M. the next day, and so on.

Keep in mind that although you might be able to influence the times at which your baby sleeps, you cannot alter his sleep needs. If he needs only eleven hours of sleep out of each twenty-four, you may be able to influence which eleven hours out of the daily cycle he spends sleeping, but you will not have much luck in trying to get him to sleep more than eleven hours.

Winding Down

A regular schedule and a mellow bedtime ritual are standard formulas from most baby sleep experts. In the half-hour or so just before bedtime, don't play tickling games or even peek-a-boo to make him laugh. These activities will over-stimulate him and get him worked up and active.

Make this routine as simple or as elaborate as you want. How does your baby like baths? If your baby finds his bath a relaxing experience, there's a natural way to get him calm and ready to drift off to sleep when he gets into his crib or your bed.

After he's had his bath and you've toweled him off, get him into his pajamas or whatever clothing he normally wears to bed. When baby wears something different to bed than he wears all day, this signals him that it's time for something different—going to sleep. He'll eventually associate his pajamas with bedtime.

Close the blinds or curtains and turn off all the lights except his night-light, if you use one. You can carry him as you perform these tasks. He'll soon learn to associate all of these activities with the fact that it's time to go to bed and go to sleep.

What's next? Perhaps a lullaby. A lullaby doesn't have to be a song about going to sleep. Any soft song will do. It might be an old childhood favorite, nursery rhyme, or popular song with a gentle rhythm and slow tempo. Choose something that you like, too; you may be singing it for a few years to come.

Smart Mama Tricks: Attitude Is Everything

If you tense up at bedtime because you're dreading the possibility that he won't go right to sleep, he'll sense your tension and react to it. If you rush because you're in a hurry to get him to sleep so you can enjoy dinner with your spouse or because you're simply eager to relax alone, you won't communicate the peacefulness and ease that you need to convey to your baby. Breathe deeply and remain calm.

Bedtime stories are popular and educational, whether you read from a book, tell him a story from memory, or make one up. Many babies fall in love with a favorite book and request it, night after night, as they get older.

When Night Is Day and Day Is Night

If your older baby remains active at night, there are a number of things you can do to help. To begin with, don't play with him when the room is dark. If he cries, hold him and soothe him, but this isn't the time for "This Little Piggy." It will take him a while to get the message, but stick with it. Don't ignore his cries, but show him that nighttime is not playtime.

Don't make the mistake of trying to keep your baby awake by day in order to get him tired enough to sleep at night. This tactic frequently backfires: Your child may become overtired and have trouble falling asleep at night. Let baby sleep during the day, but if he takes an extended nap, consider waking him up after three hours or so. As much as possible, plan car trips (errands and such) either at times when you would expect baby to be napping or just after a nap, when he is least likely to succumb to the lulling motion of the car. In other words, try not to let car trips provide an occasion for extra daytime naps.

♡ Take Care of You: Share the Load

If you're expressing milk and baby is taking a bottle, or if you're bottle-feeding formula, trade nights with your partner or take shifts. For example, you can feed the waking baby from 10:00 P.M. to 2:00 A.M. and he can do it from 2:00 A.M. to 6:00 A.M. This way, you're both assured some sleep.

Helping Baby Help Himself

Once your baby outgrows the middle-of-the-night feedings, he may still wake up. He may have a bona fide need, such as being thirsty or too warm, or he may simply have woken up to move around or roll over. This is not a problem unless he cannot get himself back to sleep again.

If your older baby does wake up during the night, what should you do? First of all, whether he is in a crib or sleeping beside you in bed, listen closely. He may wake up, make a little bit of noise as he finds himself awake at an unwanted hour, and then slowly settle down and go back to sleep. If you hear your baby making cooing noises, soft cries, or anything other than a true cry, don't go running into his room. Listen to see if he works his way back to sleep on his own. If he can't, he'll let you know—quickly!

And if he doesn't settle down quickly, then by all means attend to him. Though there's an old school of thought that advocates letting your older baby cry himself to sleep once you are sure that he's not hungry, hot or cold, in need of burping, or otherwise in discomfort, most experts disagree with this thinking. After all, something is bothering the baby, even if it is merely his inability to get back to sleep. He is seeking help of some sort, even if it is only the comfort of your presence and companionship at a time when he is awake and doesn't want to be. He can't speak and tell you what is troubling him. All he can do is cry. It's his only form of communication. Let him know you understand and are there for him.

Is It a Problem?

Before you even begin to look for advice on "fixing" a sleep problem, you first have to decide whether you or your baby even has a problem. If your nine- or twelve-month-old is sleeping for four or five hours at a time, wakes up once or twice at night to feed, and you both quickly go back to sleep, then there may not really be a problem. Especially if everyone is well rested the next day, you may not want to adjust anything to eliminate those feedings or awakenings.

Sleep Programs

As you try to decide what to do about your baby and sleep, consider what will work for you and what will work for your baby. Don't worry that you're stuck once you make your choice. If you're like most parents, you'll try a few methods, settle on one for your first child, and then find that it's completely ineffective for your second.

There are a few rules that many—but not all—of the programs share. If you don't want to go all the way with any one approach, you might start with these elements as you work out a system of your own:

- Try to put your baby down to sleep when he is drowsy but awake. This may teach him to put himself back to sleep when he wakes up.

- Establish a pre-bed ritual and try not to vary from it. Make sure it is of a reasonable length and includes books or songs that you won't be tired of for years to come.

- Get your older baby (at least four months old AND able to easily roll over and lift and move his head) attached to a baby-safe "lovey," also known as a "transitional object." The idea here is that the baby will look for the lovey when he wants to calm down. Some people do question whether you want your baby to bond with you, the mother, or with a yellow duck, but when you absolutely can't be there, lovies really come in handy.

- Don't do anything. Your baby will eventually sleep through the night—at least sometime before he's a teenager, at which point your problem will be dragging him out of bed before noon.

Ask the Experts

As with most parenting issues, there are many experts whose books you can read for help in getting your baby to sleep well. Each offers suggestions and tips to avoid challenging sleep habits and help your baby sleep all night. Choose the one that fits best with your own parenting style.

The advice from all of the experts is often quite similar, and the main difference often lies in whether or not to let the baby "cry it out."

William and Martha Sears

Authors of many bestselling parenting books, Dr. William Sears, a pediatrician, and his wife Martha, a nurse, are often seen as advocates of "attachment parenting." Their most recent offering, *The Baby Sleep Book: The Complete Guide to a Good Night's Rest for the Whole Family*, offers help for all sleep-deprived parents. This excellent resource teaches parents how to match their baby's temperament to their own lifestyle and tailor their own sleep methods accordingly.

Elizabeth Pantley

The No-Cry Sleep Solution was devised by Elizabeth Pantley, parent educator and mother of four. Pantley first teaches you about sleep and sleep safety; then has you log your baby's naps, pre-bedtime routines, and night waking into detailed charts; and from there, helps you create a customized sleep plan to help your child sleep increasingly longer stretches through the night.

Richard Ferber

If you don't like to let your baby cry, then Dr. Richard Ferber isn't for you. His revised 2006 edition of *Solve Your Child's Sleep Problems* (originally published 20 years ago) still utilizes the "cry it out" approach, but now Ferber states it's not a catch-all solution for every baby or situation. He recommends that once your baby is five to six months old and not sleeping well, you teach him to fall asleep on his own and let him cry for progressively longer periods of time before briefly checking on him.

But I Still Can't Sleep!

There may be times when you've tried all of the sleep strategies you know to get your baby to sleep, but your baby just won't sleep. Something is keeping him awake, and therefore, you are also kept up. There you are, sleepy but sleepless, frustrated, and at your wits' end. What are you going to do?

Perhaps he's simply going to be awake for a while, maybe even for several hours—but he's not crying as long as you hold him. Try to think of it as spending some more precious time with your baby (soon enough you'll wonder when he grew up so fast) and make the best of it. If you let yourself get frustrated at his wakefulness and your resultant inability to sleep, you'll only grow angry at him and become so agitated that, even when he finally does go back to sleep, you'll be unable to drift off yourself.

Better to relax and rest as best you can, perhaps in your rocking chair, with your baby in one arm and a good book in the other hand. If you can put on some soft, relaxing music without waking anyone else, go ahead and do it. Even if it doesn't do anything for your baby, you need to relax.

♡ Take Care of You: **Swap Naps with a Friend**

Find another mother you trust who has a baby of comparable age and would be willing to trade off with you. One mom watches both babies while the other mom naps.

Try to accept that there are going to be periods of wakefulness during the night in baby's early months, especially during the first weeks, and that you're going to lose sleep. He won't be up all night. Babies of that age almost never stay awake for eight-hour stretches.

Sleep Deprivation

Some additional things you can do:

- Accept that when baby is napping during the day it's more important that you nap rather than clean the house or cook a fancy dinner.
- Sit or lie down as much as possible, even when you can't sleep.
- If you're sleep-deprived due to baby being awake at night, rather than overdose on coffee to stay alert, which might keep you awake if he suddenly decides to go to sleep and give you an opportunity for a nap, rely on extra showers to wake you up and refresh you. Then you have a better chance at napping if your baby naps.
- Don't focus on how tired you are. It will only make you feel worse.

Don't let your tiredness tempt you into anything risky like lying down on the sofa with the baby on top of you and your arms around him to hold him in place or lying there with the baby wedged between you and the sofa back. No matter how tired you are, don't take such risks.

No One Is to Blame

If the baby isn't a "good sleeper," it's not that you're being a bad mother. It's not that you don't know how to get him to sleep. It's not that you're doing anything wrong or failing to do something right. The baby is simply doing what babies do: crying often, sleeping in cycles that don't conform to yours, and demonstrating perfectly normal, natural actions that are in no way the result of any failure or inadequacy on your part.

Don't blame the baby, either. Don't say, "He's not good," though you can say "He's not a good sleeper yet." (Hang on to that "yet"—it indicates hope for the future.) Sleeping patterns are not "behavior" in the sense of being "well behaved" or "badly behaved."

So do your best to calm him down, be grateful when he goes back to sleep, make sure your partner does his fair share, and get rest whenever you can. Better days—and nights—are ahead.

Chapter 8

Sex and the Mommy

Right after your baby is born, sex is probably the furthest thing from your mind. You just pushed an infant the size of a watermelon out your vagina, and you'd appreciate no one touching you down there, thank you very much. But don't worry. The feelings of love and affection will return. You and your partner do remember what life was like before the baby came, and postpartum sex will become a reality.

Cleared for Takeoff

Most doctors advise waiting until your six-week checkup before resuming sexual activity. In reality, there is no "magic" wait time. While six weeks may be just the right amount of time for one person, it may be too long or too short for you. If you feel ready before then, be sure to talk to your provider for clearance before proceeding with sex. Even after the six-week wait, know that the first several times you have sex can hurt—in some cases, a lot. The good news is that eventually things will return to normal.

When He Wants To and You Don't

Most women experience a lack of interest in sex following the birth of their baby. Hormonal changes serve to focus a new mother's attention where nature wants it, on the baby. It's a temporary condition, but combined with sleep deprivation, it can leave little room for romance.

Physically, your vaginal area may still be tender, and your scar from any episiotomy or tearing may be sensitive. You might feel just fine physically, but the memory of how much the birth hurt may still make you cringe. Your body may feel odd when you are touched, in part because the hormonal effects of breastfeeding change your skin (this can be remedied with lotion or massage oil), and also because you're being touched so much by your baby you just can't take any more.

Intimacy Instead

Intimacy doesn't mean sex. Rather, true intimacy is a matter of the mind. It's simply knowing and caring about your partner's thoughts, needs, and feelings, but mostly it's about trust. Trust that you'll be there when you're needed, trust that you'll love your partner no matter what, and trust that you can be yourself with each other.

Where there's true intimacy between a couple, sex follows naturally. Until you're both ready for physical intimacy, you can stay connected with your partner in many simple, nonsexual ways.

- Leave love notes around the house for your mate.
- Take a walk together.
- Surprise your partner with a gift. It doesn't have to be anything big, just a little way of saying, "I'm thinking of you."

- Say "I love you" and mean it.
- Go on a date. Take a deep breath and hire that babysitter. Go to your favorite restaurant or have a picnic. It's all right to talk about the baby. It might be hard to think about anything else at first. Your child is the focus of your life right now, but don't let that one topic dominate the conversation.
- Rent a funny movie and laugh together.
- Take an interest in the activities your mate enjoys.
- Give or receive a massage. A breastfeeding mom is especially prone to sore back and shoulders.
- Look your best. Often, you just need to be comfortable around your home, and sweatpants and a T-shirt are fine. On occasion, though, treat your spouse to the glamorous version of you that's usually reserved for special events.
- Write a love song or rewrite the words to an existing song. Your song can be dripping with romance or it can be funny. Or burn a CD of the songs that are special to the two of you.
- Give up some minor habit you know annoys your mate. Tapping your fingers or putting your elbows on the table might seem like minor issues, but changing your behavior out of love is a major gesture.

Heavy Petting

It may take a while for you and your partner to get back on track. In the meantime, consider alternatives to sex. Sometimes snuggling is a happy medium. You may find that this meets his need for physical companionship and meets your need for affection without actual intercourse.

However, cuddling may not always do the trick. If he is really in the mood for sex and you are not, there are still alternatives. You can consider sending him off to take a cold shower—or you could offer to shower with him and use it as a chance to take care of his needs through masturbation, with or without you. Remember to be considerate and respectful of his needs, just as you'd like him to be toward yours.

> ♡ Take Care of You: **A Little Foreplay Goes a Long Way**
>
> *Sometimes your aversion to sex can be overcome by initiating romance. There might be times when you think you are too tired, but a little kissing quickly gets you in the mood. This is fine; just let your partner know that you hold the right to bail at any time.*

Keep Talking

Through it all, communicate. Talk about everything. It's especially important to discuss your feelings before a problem develops. Talk to your partner about the fact that you don't always have matching libidos and that it may not be because of the baby. Otherwise, he may believe that the baby is taking his place in your life. He won't know this isn't the case unless you tell him.

When You Want To and He Doesn't

This scenario is less common, but it's not unheard of. Before your baby was born, your relationship with your partner took center stage. You were lovers, friends, and playmates. Now, you're Mom and Dad. For some people, it's hard to reconcile these new roles with the old ones. Some men believe that their wife's new status as a mother makes her untouchable.

Guys like that need a little reminder that their mates are still sexual beings. Are moms sexy? You bet they are. Mothers are women, not girls. They have given birth. They're fertile and sensuous. If you're ready for sex but your partner doesn't seem interested, make the first move. Most men love that. It might be just the thing he needs to jog his memory about how you became parents in the first place.

♡ Take Care of You: Time for a New Diaphragm

If you used a diaphragm prior to getting pregnant, you will require a new prescription after your baby is born. Giving birth may change the diaphragm size you require, and an ill-fitting diaphragm can lead to an unwanted pregnancy.

The Battle for the Breast

Breastfeeding and sex are not mutually exclusive. You can enjoy a sexual relationship with your partner even though you are spending much of your days and nights nursing your infant. Be aware that you may leak milk during sex; but this can be diminished or thwarted by nursing your baby (hopefully to sleep) shortly before lovemaking begins.

The Big Moment

Sometime after getting the six-week go-ahead (possibly way after, particularly, research shows, if your baby wakes frequently at night), you may find yourself having fond memories of sex, fond enough to contemplate having it again, in spite of your exhaustion. Or, more likely, you may want to try it just once to reassure yourself that everything still works, and then have no interest again for months. When you hit this point, think lubrication—and take a few other special precautions.

Relax. Some women friends may advise alcohol as a way to "get in the mood," but breastfeeding mothers need to be careful about using a glass of wine or any other alcoholic beverage to help them relax. Whenever you plan to have a drink, nurse your baby first, and allow at least one hour to pass for every alcoholic drink you consume before breastfeeding your baby again. If you feed your baby and then have two glasses of wine, you should wait at least two hours from the last drink. One final word about alcohol: Most new moms are exhausted and alcohol can send them right to sleep. Instead, ask your partner for a slow and gentle pre-coital massage.

Lubricate. Postpartum estrogen levels reduce your vagina's natural lubrication, so have a tube of the artificial stuff on hand. Astroglide is a good choice. Spermicidal jellies are another. Normal amounts of lubrication usually return after your first menstrual cycle.

Use birth control. You might need to try a different method than usual while breastfeeding. Nonchemical methods, such as condoms, diaphragms, and cervical caps, are usually safest for the breastfeeding baby.

Take the lead. Postpartum women generally prefer to be on top or to lay side-by-side with their partner (the spoon position) during intercourse. These positions let you control the amount of pressure put on your delicate perineal tissue.

Communicate. Let your husband know what you enjoy and what's just too uncomfortable right now. Don't suffer through the event. Your partner wants you to enjoy yourself. That might be a tall order the first few times, but at a minimum, you shouldn't have to be in pain. If you decide to grin and bear it, you're just going to be even more nervous about sex in the future.

Expect some milk leakage. Sexual stimulation releases oxytocin, the hormone that causes your milk ejection, or letdown, reflex. Your breasts might leak when you make love and even spray your partner in the face when you orgasm. If that's a problem (and who says it has to be?), nurse your baby before you have sex or wear a bra and nursing pads. In any case, you'll want to keep a towel handy. Those things are loaded and they might just go off.

Take your time. It's been a while, but a new mom's body is too sensitive to rush things. Dad, you've waited this long, a few more minutes won't hurt. Foreplay should be long and relaxed.

Timing Is Everything

Once you've broken the ice that first time, you'll need to find more time for romance in the future. It might sound like Mission Impossible, but you can plan for those special times with your partner. Just stay as well rested as you can and keep track of the times during the day and night when your baby is blissfully asleep. Those are your opportunities.

> ### ♡ Take Care of You: **A Night Away**
>
> *When you're ready, call your mother, your best friend, your trusted sitter, and then book a night in a nearby hotel. You'll be close enough to rush home should you be desperately needed; meanwhile, you'll have an entire uninterrupted night with your partner. You may never leave the bed.*

It can take anywhere from a few weeks to an entire year for sex to become as comfortable as it was before pregnancy. Then you'll face a whole new set of challenges. Your child is mobile. If you make love when she's awake, she will find you: They're like bloodhounds. In the meantime, remember that your life will not always involve planning when and where to have sex. Be wild. Take a chance. Sometimes the mood will strike and the timing will be off. Occasionally it will all work out perfectly. At times, you'll both wind up a bit frustrated or laughing about how everything turned out. No matter what, there's no harm in trying.

Chapter 9

Baby Health 411

She's sick! Do you call the doctor? Dash to the emergency room? Give her medicine? Or just put her back to sleep? You're the triage nurse and you have to figure it out—which isn't easy, particularly because she's still screaming. Here are some sick- and well-baby basics, from choosing a provider to surviving your child's illnesses. Remember: Confidence in your baby's health and healthcare providers is a big step toward maintaining your own sanity this year.

Picky, Picky

When deciding which pediatrician you will trust with the care of your new baby, let's start with some things that you should *not* do.

- Don't just pick a doctor from the phone book or from a list provided by your insurance company.
- Don't pick simply whoever is "on-call" when your baby is born.
- Don't go to a pediatrician that someone else likes unless you ask (and agree with) what they like about the doctor.
- Don't go to a doctor just because the office is in a convenient location.

Choose a pediatrician *before* your baby is born so that if anything goes wrong in the early stages, you will know who is taking care of your baby and advising you on medical decisions that you must make. Choosing the right doctor may mean avoiding unnecessary tests or treatments from a provider who is overly aggressive or, on the flip side, avoiding a doctor who misses something important because of an inappropriate "wait-and-see" attitude. Beyond the medical emergency concerns, there are well-baby care issues. Some pediatricians are more holistically oriented, some more by-the-book Western medicine. Some have strict rules regarding vaccination schedules; others are more flexible. Decide what's important to you and interview potential doctors accordingly.

Friend or Foe

The best way to find a new pediatrician is to get recommendations from friends or family members. But always find out *why* they like their doctor. Is it simply because the office is efficient and they can get in and out quickly? Or is it because they always get an antibiotic when they want one? Make sure that you're comfortable with the reason they like the pediatrician, and that this reason has something to do with being an educated and competent doctor (not a personal preference for the way the waiting room is decorated). The same applies when a person recommends against a doctor.

Once you've narrowed down your choices, phone the pediatrician's office and schedule a "new parent" interview with the doctor. Some offices charge for this, but most offer them free of charge. Realize that a busy pediatric practice is just that, busy, and try not to take too much of the doctor's time (particularly if it's free). Be prepared with your list of questions. Consider your own expectations: Do you want to always talk to the doctor when you call for advice, and not have to speak with a nurse? Do you expect these calls to last fifteen or thirty minutes? Find out if the doctor agrees with your positions on important matters, like breastfeeding, antibiotic overuse, circumcision, and so on. If not, is she at least flexible and willing to help you do things the way you want?

 Smart Mama Tricks: **First Thing in the Morning**

When your baby is sick, don't wait until the last minute to make an appointment. The earlier you call once your pediatrician's office opens in the morning, the sooner you'll get an appointment. If you wait until late in the day, you might be asked to wait until the next day, even for a problem that has been going on for several days.

Ask the front desk staff about office protocol, such as:

- Whether they accept your insurance
- Office hours
- Wait times
- Whether you will always be able to see your pediatrician (if it's a group practice)

- Last-minute urgent care visits
- How far ahead you must schedule well-baby appointments
- Hospital affiliations
- Whether someone is available on-call after hours

While you're questioning the front desk personnel, you can gauge your general comfort level with them, as well.

You Can Always Change Your Mind

Don't fret if you are having a seemingly impossible time making a decision. Even with recommendations and a good prenatal visit, it still takes a few "real-world" visits to find out if you've found the "right" pediatrician.

 Smart Mama Tricks: **The Rule of Fridays**

If you have a medical concern on a Friday, call the pediatrician. Chances are, the condition will worsen over the weekend and you'll find yourself stuck for hours in the waiting room of the E.R. or the local Urgent Care clinic. Save yourself the worry, time, and headache and contact your baby's doctor right away during office hours.

It could be that there is a policy you didn't know about, or maybe the doctor was simply on her best behavior for the "interview." If you later encounter problems with your pediatrician or her office and you can't resolve them, start the process over and look for another one.

Call the Doctor

It seems like a no-brainer, but many new moms actually hesitate to phone their pediatrician with concerns. They think, "I'm being paranoid," "She's tired of hearing from me over every sniffle," "The nurse is going to lecture me again on how The Fever Is Our Friend," etc. Here's some news for you: That's what the doctor is there for. That's what you pay her for. If anything about your infant's health concerns you, follow your gut and call your doctor. They see new parents like you every day. If there is truly nothing wrong with your child, then you have set your mind at ease—which is a good thing. And many pediatricians know that "mother's intuition" often rings true. However, if you ever feel like you are getting "attitude" from the doctor or her office staff, find another physician with whom you feel comfortable. This is the baby's health you're talking about. You are in charge.

Always call the pediatrician if you observe any of the following:

- A rectal temperature of 100.4° Fahrenheit or above (when the baby is less than three months old)
- A temperature above 101° Fahrenheit (from three to six months)
- A temperature above 103° Fahrenheit (after six months)
- Trouble breathing

- Fussiness that doesn't improve when you hold him, especially if he also has a fever, poor appetite, or other symptoms
- Projectile vomiting or vomiting up a dark green substance
- Vomiting and/or diarrhea that is causing dehydration
- Bloody diarrhea
- Poor appetite, not eating well
- Excessive sleeping or difficulty waking him up
- Problems breastfeeding to the point at which you feel you may need to supplement

There aren't specific guidelines about when to call if your older infant has a fever, so even if your seven-month-old has just a low-grade fever of 101° and you are concerned, call your pediatrician.

Before you phone the doctor, have the following information on hand:

- Your doctor's name (if it's a group practice)
- Your baby's temperature (even if it's normal)
- A list of symptoms, starting with the ones that concern you most, and an estimate of their duration
- What you've done to address these symptoms
- The phone number of a pharmacy that is open, convenient, and accepts your insurance
- Your baby's weight at his last checkup (in case your doctor wants to check on the dosage of a medication)

You should also trust your instincts and call any other time that you think your baby is ill and you need help.

Help Him Help You

You will make lots of visits to your pediatrician's office during your infant's first year of life, for well-baby checkups as well as sick calls. Knowing what to expect can help you make the most of these visits.

Don't waste what time you have in the doctor's office. A fussy baby and sibling control are two of many possible distractions that can lead you astray. Prepare a list of questions to ensure you don't forget anything important.

Well Visits

At each well-baby visit, in addition to a standard history and physical, your pediatrician should have your baby's height, weight, and head circumference recorded and plotted on a growth chart to make sure that he is growing well. The exam should also include an eye exam, and a hip check to evaluate for developmental dislocation.

Sick Visits

Don't assume that a doctor can tell what is wrong with a sick baby just by the physical exam. In reality, the history (or story of the child's illness) can be even more important. Suppose your baby has a cough and runny nose. If he is eating and drinking well, isn't too fussy, isn't having trouble breathing, and the symptoms just started yesterday, then he likely just has a cold and doesn't need any antibiotics. If, however, he has had two weeks of symptoms that are now worsening and has begun to have a fever, he might have a sinus infection and may need antibiotics. Both cases would probably have the same physical exam; but your description of the illness would get him the right treatment.

Some possible questions that you should be prepared to answer during a sick visit:

- How long has your child been sick?
- What are all of his symptoms?
- When are the symptoms worse?
- Has he been around anyone else who's been sick?
- What medications have you been giving him?
- Why do you think he hasn't been getting better?
- What are you most worried about with this illness?

When doctors, nurses, and other people working in the ER do not have specific training in caring for pediatric patients, your child can be misdiagnosed, overtreated, or have to undergo too many unnecessary tests. Avoid these potential problems by trying to call your pediatrician before you head to the ER, unless it is a true emergency. Once you arrive, you might also ask what type of pediatric training and experience the ER staff has, ask them to call your pediatrician to review the diagnosis and treatment plan, or ask for a transfer to a facility that has board-certified emergency medicine physicians or pediatric specialists.

Common Illnesses

Although you'll worry if your child gets sick a lot, remember that the average child gets six to eight upper-respiratory-tract infections, such as colds and sore throats, and two to three episodes of diarrhea each year, especially if he's in day care.

Colds and Sinus Infections

The most frequent cause of a runny nose in younger kids is the common cold. Like most other viral infections, there is no treatment for the common cold. You often just have to treat your baby's symptoms until he gets over them on his own.

Cold symptoms typically begin with a clear runny nose, low-grade fever, and a cough. Over the next few days the symptoms may worsen, with a higher fever and worsening cough. The runny nose might become yellow or green before going away over the next one to two weeks. This is the normal pattern for a cold and does not mean that your child has a sinus infection or needs antibiotics. Of course, if your child is very fussy, is not eating or drinking, or has trouble breathing, then see your doctor.

To help your infant feel better, you might use saline nasal drops and suctioning with a nasal aspirator to clear your infant's nose, a cool-mist humidifier or vaporizer, and, on advice of your pediatrician, an age-appropriate dose of a pain and fever reducer and/or a cold and cough medicine. Remember that infants and children should not take aspirin because of the risk of Reye's syndrome, a life-threatening liver disorder.

♡ Take Care of You: **Lighten Your Load**

Taking care of a baby is hard; taking care of a sick baby is harder. Admit it and don't try to carry on with your normal activities. Ask for help from family and friends if you need it.

While a yellow or green runny nose is typically caused by a common cold, if the infection lingers for more than ten to fourteen days and is worsening, or if the child has a high fever for more than three or four days and appears ill, then he may really have a sinus infection that requires antibiotics.

Ear Infections

You may suspect an ear infection when your baby starts pulling on his ears, but unless there are other symptoms, like a fever or irritability, the ears are usually okay. More typically, an ear infection develops a few days or weeks after having a cold. A child will experience ear pain, irritability, fever, and a decreased appetite. Although symptoms sometimes go away without treatment, doctors still commonly prescribe antibiotics, especially for babies under the age of twelve to twenty-four months.

Vomiting and Diarrhea

For most parents, diarrhea and vomiting are among the more distressing symptoms of illness. Yet both of these symptoms are generally easy to treat. When caused by a virus (as they typically are), your goal is to prevent dehydration. If the only symptom is diarrhea and your child is either nursing or eating and drinking well, you can often continue his regular diet and, if he's not nursing anymore, give a few ounces of an oral rehydration solution each time he has diarrhea.

If your child also vomits a lot and can't keep down fluids, becomes more dehydrated, or if you're not sure what to do, call your doctor. To be safe, see your doctor if your baby has persistent vomiting for more than twenty-four hours or has other serious symptoms that concern you.

Surviving Your Baby's Sick Days (and Nights)

Clear your calendar and put away the "to do" list. If you work, call in sick. Given the amount of sleep you're probably getting, this is not a lie.

Your baby will want to be held most of the time. When he actually does fall asleep somewhere other than in your arms, you'll need to lie down yourself and rest. You'll be getting a lot less sleep at night when your baby is sick, and will probably be fighting a bug yourself.

Use Your Energy Wisely

Don't clean, don't cook, and don't do laundry (except for anything that's been pooped or thrown-up upon). Expect your baby to regress a stage. A baby who has been eating solids may only want to nurse; a baby who gave up his bottle for a cup a month ago may want his bottle again. Don't fight it—let him have what he wants now.

Your baby may wake several times a night, sometimes for hours. Don't pace the floor in the dark, bored and frustrated that you can't put him down and go back to sleep yourself. Discover late-night television. Find a trashy show that in your exhausted state of mind strikes you as funny. Or make a nest of towels on the floor and lie down with your baby. This way, your bed won't get covered by snot or vomit, and maybe you'll both get some sleep.

Use the telephone. Call your mother and cry to her. Call a far-away friend and tell her about how hard it all is. Call your nearby friends and tell them how miserable you are (maybe some of them will offer to drop off a meal).

Remember: Even though your baby is up all night crying, even though every sheet and blanket in the house needs a good washing, even though the only thing that calms him down is skipping up and down the hall—this will pass and you will sleep again.

Chapter 10

Your Parenting Village

For thousands of years, human beings lived in extended-family groups or villages, and shared knowledge and parenting chores. Today's moms, especially those who opt out of the workforce and parent full time, often find themselves alone all day with a baby in their arms and no idea what to do with themselves. No adult conversation? No other baby/parent duos to share with and learn from? Feel like you're going stir crazy? Time to create a supportive twenty-first-century parenting village of your own.

The Grandparents

Shortly after the birth of your babe, help will probably arrive in the form of family, your parents or in-laws, or perhaps a sister or aunt or cousin. Family is complicated. This may be actually helpful or incredibly difficult, depending on the relationship you share. In these days of frequent relocations and small nuclear families, grandparents can be life saving. In a perfect world, grandparents are a source of invaluable advice and support. In addition to raising their own kids, they had years of experience dealing with all the things that help a family run smoothly. Ideally, that would mean that if you have a problem, you could ask one of your baby's grandparents and get some useful advice. Some families are actually like this!

Unwanted Advice

In many families, things are more complex. Instead of getting helpful advice, you and your partner might be criticized for the way you do things. Or you may get advice that goes against the way you've chosen to raise your children, leading to hard feelings when you choose not to follow it. Some grandparents take anything you do differently as a direct condemnation of the way they parented you. Understanding why this happens and trying to avoid miscommunications can help to support a healthy relationship between your own family and all of the grandparents.

> ♡ Take Care of You: **To Each Your Own**
>
> *In general, when dealing with conflicts, each person should speak with his or her own biological parents. You have a long history with your own folks, and this may help you to avoid your in-laws viewing you as the bad guy.*

There was a time when doctors actively discouraged mothers from breastfeeding and recommended that they not hold their baby very much because it might spoil him. Parents also were advised to start solid and table foods a lot earlier than now. Even childproofing, car seats, and other safety measures weren't widely supported when many of you were kids.

While mothers and mothers-in-law often come to stay for a week or so after the birth, some new moms feel more inclined to entertain them as guests, rather than to accept their help. If this is you, limit the number of visitors who come to call during the first few weeks after your baby arrives. If you have a hard time saying no, ask your partner to screen your calls or simply say, "I'd like to have you over once things settle down a bit. I appreciate your patience and look forward to seeing you."

Because today's grandparents raised their children using different advice, it's no surprise that their recommendations are a bit (or a lot) different from the methods you use now. Is your two-month-old not sleeping through the night? Don't be surprised if a grandparent tells you to feed him cereal to help him sleep. Or maybe your mother will insist that your baby doesn't need to breastfeed or that she should be put to sleep on her stomach.

You can try to explain that those things aren't recommended anymore, but it's hard to do this without making grandparents feel that they did things wrong. Instead of dismissing or criticizing a grandparent's advice, try to explain why recommendations have changed—for example, that a baby who sleeps on her stomach is at higher risk for SIDS.

Because grandparents can have such a positive role in the life of your baby, it's worth it to try to maintain a healthy relationship. That can be hard, though, especially with all of the added stress and anxiety that a new baby brings.

Be specific about what your needs are. Do you need help watching your baby? Or would you rather spend more time with your baby but need some extra help around the house in order to do this? Try to ensure that grandparents have the chance to visit and spend as much time with their grandchild as they'd like.

Meanwhile, in this as in all aspects of parenting, remember the adage: Fight the fights worth fighting. Let the little things go.

♡ Take Care of You: "Educating" Grandparents

If your baby's grandparents on either side of the family are having a hard time understanding how parenting, medical, and safety advice have changed, consider inviting them to one of your baby's well visits to his pediatrician, or to your parenting class if you're attending one. That way, they can hear that advice firsthand, ask questions, and learn to better support your methods of raising your baby.

Extended Family

Brothers, sisters, aunts, uncles—enlist help and join forces with every family member you can. If you have children at the same time as one of your sibs and live close by, you can share babysitting, outings, birthdays, and the like.

Friends with Kids

A good friend is never worth more than now—when you are in such a state of flux adjusting to your first year with baby. The changes that you go through physically and emotionally demand the ear of a friend. Though your relationships with old friends have changed over the years, you may still have some of them in your life. If so, you're lucky. But you also need to find new friends with babies. Moms just like you.

Eventually, you'll need to get out of the house. Your world will begin to revolve less solely around your newborn and more around your new life as a whole. This change comes at different times for everyone. You may feel like getting out and being social at six weeks postpartum. Or you may wish to wait a few months.

Support Groups

Remember the room full of big bellies and nervous, expectant faces in your old pregnancy classes? You were all in the same boat then, and chances are, you're all in the same boat now. But instead of gathering together in the same classroom once a week, you're all probably sitting alone in your living rooms with babies on your laps. Before the birth of your baby, you were probably too focused on your own impending life changes to focus on other couples and forming new friendships. But there is no better time than the present. Phone your instructor and ask if you can arrange a class reunion. You can all swap childbirth experiences and coo over each other's babies. Who knows? Some of you may hit it off and form a mother's group or play group that could last for years to come.

Lactation Support Groups

A roomful of new moms breastfeeding their infants with an expert consultant on hand—there aren't many safer, friendlier, or more supportive first outings than this. Often, your local hospital, birthing center, or La Leche League organization offers these weekly gatherings free of charge. Whether you are having breastfeeding issues or everything is going just fine, a lactation support meeting is an excellent choice for finding new friends and support.

Post Partum Yoga or Stroller Exercise Classes

Once you're gotten the okay from your provider, you can think about working out again. A bonus: these parent-child classes are filled with like-minded moms with babies of differing ages and stages. You can hook up with a parent of a child several months older, who can provide needed experience and advice, or with parents of infants the same age as yours. Ask a potential new friend if she'd like to meet you for a walk outside of class hours. Your babies may snooze happily to the motion in their slings, front packs, or jog strollers while you enjoy some great conversation, exercise, and fresh air.

Parenting Classes

Check the adult education department of your local school district or the child development department of your community college for "babes-in-arms" parenting classes. Not only will you learn a great deal about infant and child care, but you will get to hang out with your baby and meet other parent/infant duos at the same time. Many informal parenting groups form out of these classes once the semester or program concludes.

The Local Park

If you're lucky enough to have a nice park with a playground nearby (or even if you have to drive a bit), drop by and visit, even though your child may not be old enough to enjoy the play structures yet. It's a great place to meet other moms.

Local Mothers'/Fathers' Groups

Mothers' groups can be such a boon. You've got women to talk to and babies to play with—who could ask for more? These organized groups are designed to help boost your confidence as a new mom and educate you on issues that you may not have thought about since becoming a mother.

♡ Take Care of You: **Don't Reinvent the Wheel**

These new mommy friends are your resources. Ask them questions. You will get as many different answers as you have friends. Read parenting and baby books (when you can) with many viewpoints. You are your best filter. Let all of this knowledge sift through you; then make informed choices based on your insight, experience, and the personality and individual needs of your child. You'll know what's right for you and your family.

Some obvious places to look for a new-mothers' group would be from your local birth network. Or try the hospitals or birth centers in your area. There may also be community-based programs, so check the paper. Ask other moms if they know of any in your area. Some groups are formed from other groups; for instance, your local La Leche League may have a new mothers' discussion/playgroup outside of their regular meetings. Check with local preschools to see if they run formal or informal groups for new moms and babies.

This is a great way to get out and meet other moms, while learning about taking care of yourself and your baby. These friendships that are built around your children are wonderful in many respects. You have an instant bond. And your baby gains instant playmates as he gets older and begins to play near other children.

♡ Take Care of You: **Making the Break**

Sometimes leaving a playgroup really isn't about anyone but you and your family. If you simply can't find the time or energy for playgroup, don't sweat it. Your baby will have other opportunities to play, and you will make your own opportunities to have time with other adults. But don't burn your bridges; exchange info with some mommies to set playdates when you have the time.

Moms' Group Bonuses

Once you've found your tribe, large or small, enjoy it to the fullest. Events and ideas will evolve as your needs and the needs of your children change. You may start out meeting at a different person's house each week while the babies sit in your arms or do tummy-time on blankets on the floor. Or if the weather is nice, you might meet for long walks together, followed by a picnic lunch. Then, as the babies start crawling or walking, you may choose to visit a local park for some playtime. You can plan occasional "field trips" to a zoo or aquarium.

The Meal Cooperative

Cooking meals is challenging and time-consuming (using the stove or chopping vegetables with a baby in a sling or pack is hazardous at best).

Some moms' groups opt for a monthly cook-a-thon, either all together or separately in their own kitchens. They "power cook" many servings of each meal to split up and freeze. Others rotate Saturday-night dinner preparation, where one family cooks a large meal for all the other families. The dinner can be picked up, delivered, or shared by all at one place.

If these cooking options seems unwieldy, even something as simple as a recipe exchange of quick and healthy meals can be a boon to everyone.

The Babysitting Cooperative

Once you've gotten to know your friends and their babies well and have established a strong level of trust, consider trading off babysitting duties to give each couple a well-deserved date-night or just some "me-time" for you alone. Sometimes it's easier to have your friend and her baby come to babysit at your house, so your child is in his own environment. Some children are happy being dropped off at their friend's house. Just take a deep breath, keep goodbyes brief and upbeat, and keep your cell phone on.

Mom's Night Out and Family Days

Now we're talking! All of the moms meet for dinner, to see a show, or just to hang out at someone's house without babies, while their partners or caregivers watch the children.

Family Day presents a way to get everyone together on a weekend—dads and sibs included. Picnics, potlucks, and barbecues at the park are popular—that way no one has the pressure of hosting everyone at their home. Some groups alternate Mom's Nights and Family Nights every other month.

The Annual Group Vacation

If all of the families in the group get along well, try a yearly summer vacation, perhaps a camping trip to keep things within budget, or a beach vacation. As some families relocate over the years, this holiday provides a wonderful way for everyone to stay in touch and reconnect every year.

Online Friends

The Internet has done a lot for parenting and pregnancy. As we have moved away from our families and friends and started families of our own, feelings of isolation can creep in. Not only can the Internet and its associated technologies help us stay in touch with our families, but it can help us meet friends we'd never have met any other way. This can help create a bond between women who may never have met otherwise. It brings you together in a safe place to ask questions. There are a myriad of Web sites dedicated to parenting and motherhood, and they're often great places to ask the embarrassing questions about baby poop or bloody discharge as your periods return.

Chapter 11

Mobile Mom

Babies are portable. They are easy to carry, will sleep just about anywhere, and don't beg to stop at every McDonald's. Take advantage of it while you can and take your baby on the road with you. Go out often; your baby will thrive on exposure to new sights, sounds, and smells, and you'll keep yourself from going nuts. You once had a life outside the house and you can continue to do so.

Baby-to-Go

Babies love to be held, and adults love to hold babies. But parents have busy lives and can't sit around holding their babies all day, no matter how much they'd like to. For this reason, parents need a way to hold their babies while getting other things done, from vacuuming the floor to talking on the phone. Luckily, many different types of baby carriers can help you hold your baby and keep your hands free for other tasks. And there are a plethora of strollers, joggers, and car seats to keep baby safe and secure on the go.

Slings and Front Packs

Slings are pieces of fabric that hold your baby on your body, distributing the weight from shoulder to hip. They can be used from the newborn period until your child weighs about thirty-five pounds. There are several different types of holds that can be used with the slings, depending on your preference and the baby's age.

There are a myriad of sling styles available. Some are better for moms with shoulder issues, for example, or for moms who wish to breastfeed in them. Some are adjustable, and others come in different sizes. Visit *www.TheBabyWearer.com* or *www.Peppermint.com* for sling choices, reviews, and more information.

Smart Mama Tricks: Nurse in the Sling

Breastfeeding in a sling is a wonderful, discreet option. Once you get the hang of it, you can also learn to nurse while moving around. This can be a lifesaver if you find yourself running errands and need to feed a hungry baby in public.

Front packs are just what they sound like: backpacks for the front of your body. There are many varieties available, perhaps the Baby Bjorn being the best known, all with different systems of snaps and buttons to help you position your baby. Your baby can face either inward, which is recommended until she can hold her own head up, or outward.

The main complaint about front packs and slings is that they can be difficult to learn to use. However, once you do, they make life with baby so much easier. Ask your friends if you can try on their carriers or slings before selecting one for your personal use.

 Smart Mama Tricks: One for Dad, Too

Slings and other carriers are not just for moms. Many dads love using these items to hold their babies and bond with them. Consider buying two slings or carriers—one for Mom and one for Dad—to account for body size differences or just for convenience.

Backpacks

Baby backpacks are a more comfortable option for the bigger, heavier baby, as they place less stress on your back. Make sure your child can sit up and fully control his own head before you place him in one of these carriers. Most backpacks have an internal or external frame support system, although some are soft carriers, similar to some slings and front packs. Make sure there is a strap system to ensure that baby does not fall out. The amount of additional storage space for water, snacks, diapers and the like, varies from pack to pack.

Carrying the baby behind you makes chores such as cooking and shopping much easier, particularly if you have a baby who likes to reach out and touch everything. On the other hand, it's hard to know exactly what baby is up to back there. Carry a small mirror so you can periodically check on baby. If you have a hair-puller, you'll have to find a way to distract him at times, such as attaching a toy to the pack within his reach.

Smart Mama Tricks: Stability Matters

Look for a backpack with a wide, stable "kickstand" base, so you can stand it up relatively safely while you take baby in and out of the pack or when you take the pack on and off. Be wary of leaving baby to nap in the backpack on the ground or using the backpack as a high chair. He may wake—or squirm—and tip himself over.

Some packs come with bells and whistles such as sun-and-rain hoods, detachable daypacks, and hydration system compatibility. Decide what you want your backpack for—jaunts to the grocery store or long hikes into the outback. The Web site *www.childcarriers.com* is a good place to start your search.

Strollers and Joggers

Strollers for infants should fully recline. Some moms opt for the infant car seat/stroller combo, where the car seat can be detached from its base in the car and then snapped directly into the stroller. Once your baby can sit upright without slumping, you can use other strollers. Umbrella strollers are generally inexpensive, small, lightweight, and foldable; although they're not the sturdiest strollers, you can easily store one in the car for emergencies.

Jogging or off-road strollers are the SUVs of baby transport. These are great for long walks out of doors or on unpaved trails. Some of them are too large or unwieldy for shopping, and with their non-swivel front wheels are difficult to maneuver in tight spaces. Hybrids are becoming more popular, where you can lock or unlock the front wheel or wheels, depending on whether you are jogging (and want the stroller to track straight with minimal effort) or shopping (and need the extra maneuverability). Some jog strollers even come with shock absorbers for use over rough dirt tracks. Others convert from bike trailers into strollers.

 Smart Mama Tricks: **Try Before You Buy**

If you plan to transport your stroller or jogger by car, check it out in person before you purchase. Some fold down and collapse more easily than others, and you want to make sure it fits in your vehicle before you buy.

Check out the restraining system. The stroller or jogger should have a crotch strap and waist belts that connect to form a "T" at the very least. Some have five-point harnesses, much like that of your car seat, for extra security. Make sure your infant can't slip through leg loops that are too large for him. Test the brakes (yes, there should be brakes), and press gently down on the handles (the stroller should not easily tip over backward). Along those lines, resist hanging a heavy purse or diaper bag from the handles of a lightweight stroller—it will tip right over, and your baby could get tangled in the straps and injured. Use the under-the-seat storage for that purpose.

Again, decide what you will primarily use your stroller or jogger for before you make your choice. Do you want a simple umbrella stroller for use at the mall, or do you need a tricked-out baby jogger with full sun canopy, rain fly, and lots of storage for long runs at the park? Do you need a single stroller, or a double or a triple to carry multiples or siblings? The Web site *www.joggingstroller.com* has a handy breakdown of strollers/joggers by type of use.

Car Seats

Shopping for a car seat, with so many different brands and types available, can be overwhelming at best. There are different basic guidelines to follow depending on the car you drive and the type of seat you're looking for. The AAP states there is no "safest" or "best" car seat. You will find many brands and styles of seats that fit the guidelines, so in the end your choice comes down to personal preference. Just be sure to read the manufacturer's instructions so that you install and use the seat correctly, and make sure that the car seat actually fits in your vehicle by trying it out before you buy.

Car seats have always been hard to use, and most experts estimate that 85 percent of parents use them incorrectly. LATCH (Lower Anchors and Tethers for Children) is a new system that is installed in newer cars and car seats to make them much easier to install and use. Schedule a car seat checkup with a trained professional. Locate one near you at *www.seatcheck.org* or 1-866-SEAT-CHECK.

Infant-Only Carriers

Your first car seat will probably be an infant-only seat. This seat is designed for young infants and the rear-facing position that is safest for them. (Infants should be rear-facing until they weigh twenty pounds and are twelve months old.) One of the best features of an infant-only seat is that after installing a detachable base into the back seat of your car, you can just snap the seat into the base when you are ready to go. Then, when you reach your destination, you may detach the seat and use it as a carrier to transport your baby—which works especially well when you've just driven home, your baby is fast asleep, and you'd like to carry him into the house without waking him up. Most infant seats are solely for babies under twenty pounds.

Convertible Car Seats

"Convertible" means this seat can be used both in the rear-facing and forward-facing positions, accommodating newborns, infants, and most toddlers. These seats are generally okay until a child weighs about forty pounds. There are even some with higher weight limits that can be used as a belt-positioning booster seat for children up to sixty-five to eighty pounds. While this means that you might be able to use just one car seat until your child is three years old (and therefore buy only one), a convertible seat might not fit your newborn well and it can't be used as a carrier.

Car Seat Positioning

Although it may depend on how many other kids you have seated in the car and where the seat fits best, in almost all cases your baby will be safest in the middle of the back seat. In addition to keeping him away from side-impact collisions, it protects him from any danger from side air bags. Rear-facing car seats cannot be used in a seat with an air bag—meaning they don't belong in the front passenger seat.

The Well-Stocked Diaper Bag

For some new moms, leaving the house requires an arsenal of supplies in an enormous diaper bag, which can tip the scales at up to ten pounds. (Add baby to this, plus your own postpartum pounds, and you'll feel like you're carrying the equivalent of a Great Dane everywhere you go.) As your baby grows, so will your provisions, to include toys, several varieties of snacks and drinks, and perhaps a backpack, stroller, or jogger.

The more comprehensive your diaper bag, the less you'll end up missing or buying on the road. Use your judgment, however. If the majority of your trips are to run errands or pick up older siblings, you may not need everything on this list. Pack the less-used items in a separate bag to keep with you for day trips and overnights. Pre-pack in advance to prevent last-minute rushing—that's when you forget the essentials.

- Diapers (at least four)
- A refillable pack of baby wipes
- Diaper-rash ointment
- Plastic bags (for dirty diapers, dirty clothes, partially eaten food, etc.)
- Light blanket (to cover your baby or to use as a play mat)
- Waterproof changing pad or rubberized sheet
- Cloth diaper (for burping and general cleanup)
- Baby's sun hat
- Sunscreen (for babies over six months)
- Bottles and formula, if you're not nursing exclusively
- Food for your older baby (Cheerios, etc.)
- A snack for yourself
- Water bottle (for Mom to drink and for cleanups)
- A change of clothes for your baby
- An extra shirt for yourself
- Extra breast pads, if you use them
- Travel pack of tissues
- A few toys or rattles
- Paperback book or magazine for you (in case baby naps and you'd like to relax and read)
- Cell phone

Some moms don't feel comfortable without carrying everything on this list and more. Others tuck a clean diaper and wipes in their purse and they're off. After several trips out and about, you'll know what you need and pack accordingly.

Where To, Mama?

Exactly where you go with your baby depends a lot upon his temperament, your comfort level, and what you both enjoy. Some babies will sit happily in a restaurant for hours. Others start to scream the minute you walk in the door. Babies may react differently on different days, leaving you wondering, "But he loved the museum last week. Why is he wailing now?" And you'll start to know your baby's fussy times of the day—when he's tired and would rather be napping, for example.

On the Town

Infants don't much care where they're going when they go out, but moms tend to feel a little aimless without a destination. There are several destinations available to most of us only a walk or short drive away.

- **Stores** are great places to take babies. Furniture stores and bookstores are filled with brightly colored objects of various shapes and people who love to smile at babies. Doors designed for wheelchair access are also stroller-friendly.
- **Go grocery shopping.** Your infant car seat may be designed to clip safely to the seat of a shopping cart, or you can place it inside the basket. Perhaps your local grocery store has special carts with built-in

infant seats. (You may want to clean it with a baby wipe.) You can also shop with your baby in a front pack or sling, or, if you're only purchasing a few things, wheel him in his stroller. If your baby is eating finger foods, try the free samples, or ask for a slice of a soft fruit.

Smart Mama Trick: In-Car Emergency Kit

Keep a small bag of extras permanently in the car, for the times you forget to restock the wipes in the diaper bag or when you forget the diaper bag altogether. Include at least the following: an extra outfit, two diapers, and a small Baggie of wipes.

- Go to the **mall**, indoor or outdoor. Talk to your baby about all the things you see. Admire the fountains and window shop. (You don't have to actually buy anything.) Malls also get bonus points as a parent/baby destination because they often have clean bathrooms—some, in upscale department stores, border on luxurious.
- Visit your local **farmer's market**—a hub of stimulating sights and sounds for baby. Remember to take along a large shoulder bag or a stroller with lots of storage space where you can stow your bags of produce.
- Consider a day at a **museum**. Call ahead and confirm that the museum you are considering allows a baby backpack or a stroller. (Some don't at all; some do on certain days.) Front-carriers and slings can pretty much go anywhere. When your baby is ready to eat, pick

a bench in front of a painting you really like; if you're nursing, switch paintings when you switch breasts.

Dining Out

Take yourself out to breakfast, lunch, or dinner as often as you can when your baby is in the "luggage" stage (i.e., you can set her down anywhere and she doesn't move). Until your baby is eating solids, you don't even have to worry about selecting a child-friendly restaurant. You actually can eat at a restaurant that has tablecloths (but go early, it'll be less crazy and more fun). Become a regular at a favorite restaurant; you may find your baby "adopted" by the staff, who greet her by name. If your baby is sleeping in her car seat, you may be able to safely tuck her under the table for a while. If your baby is hungry and you're nursing, settle her in to feed; just order a meal that's not too hard to eat with one hand (choose the sandwich over the pasta)—and avoid hot soup or coffee.

 Smart Mama Tricks: **Highchair Alert**

Always inspect the restaurant highchair before you place your older baby inside. Many eateries have old chairs that don't have straps or a divider to go between the child's legs, making it possible for babies of any age to slide out underneath the tray and straight off the chair. Although his head will likely catch in the opening before he tumbles to the floor, that in itself can be a harrowing occurrence for both Mom and babe.

Once your child can join you in a meal, pick a restaurant that caters to families. If your child is noisy, the other diners won't care as much and you won't be interrupting romantic dates. The restaurant staff will be used to spills, and the other children around will entertain your baby.

Restaurants with outdoor seating are ideal. There's more for your child to look at, and many babies are easily distracted by passersby. More important, the sounds of your baby fussing or crying are not so distinct as they would be inside the restaurant.

Au Cinema

Sometimes, infants will relax on your lap or in a sling, breast- or bottle-feeding and cuddling for an entire show. If you're lucky and arrive at naptime, you might be able to nurse your baby to sleep just in time for the feature to begin.

If you worry that your baby will cry during the show, take heart. Some movie theaters have special mom/baby showings once a month or once a week—crying is expected and understood. Other cinemas have "crying rooms" inside the regular auditorium where you can sit or stand or walk around while comforting your wailing baby and not miss the show. Crying rooms tend to be sticky, to say the least, and the volume is extra loud (so that you can hear over your crying infant), so be prepared.

Breastfeeding in Public

Many breastfeeding-friendly shopping malls, restaurants, and theme parks offer family lounges where you can feed your child in a private and comfortable setting. While these areas are often welcome, you're never required to use any special place for breastfeeding. You have a right to nurse your child wherever you are allowed to be. However, some women are a little self-conscious about nursing in public, and for them, family lounges can be a godsend.

If you're more comfortable nursing in relative privacy, here are a few other places to try:

- A corner restaurant booth with your back to the room
- In a parking lot in your car
- A department store fitting room
- The back pew or child nursery at church
- The back row at a matinee
- A quiet aisle at the bookstore or library

It's probably best that you try to make nursing as private as possible. With experience, you'll learn which options provide you with enough privacy and comfort to breastfeed successfully.

Chapter 12

Traveling Babe

Who says you can't travel once you have children? If anything, your experience will be richer and your children will learn to enjoy life right alongside you. If you used to take a trip every summer, by all means, continue to do so. Don't forget: Normalization is the name of the game, and this is your new normal.

What to Bring

You've been dying for a vacation, some well-earned rest and relaxation. Be forewarned, the family vacation is not quite the restful trip you were accustomed to before you had children. You still have to take care of all of baby's needs, the diapers, the feeding, the crying, the napping. However, if you're staying in a hotel, at least you're not cleaning the house, making the beds, washing the dishes, and cooking. That's a plus.

And exposing your child to new places and new sights is a reward in itself. The family vacation is a time-honored tradition that will awaken old memories and help you create fabulous new ones, as well.

You'll develop your own packing list eventually, but here's a start.

- Car seat
- Stroller

- Baby clothes (more than you think, as you may go through several outfits a day when they get wet or soiled)
- Food for trip, including powdered formula and water if you're bottle-feeding
- Diapers and wipes (bring enough for two days; buy the rest at your destination)
- A favorite toy
- "New" toy for the trip
- Lovey, if she has one
- Portable crib, sheets, favorite blanket
- Portable highchair
- CDs of baby's favorite music if you'll be traveling by car
- Babyproofing gadgets (If your baby is crawling, babyproof at least one room at your destination, or it won't be much of a vacation for you. Bring a pack of outlet covers and a few cabinet locks.)
- Your medical insurance card and doctor's phone number
- First aid kit
- Scotch tape (endless, nondestructive entertainment for toddlers)
- Sunscreen

 Smart Mama Tricks: **The Big One**

Take that "big" vacation before your child is crawling or eating solid foods. It will be the easiest family vacation for a while.

Traveling by Car

If you're going on a long car ride, try to plan the trip around your baby's regular sleep schedule. Figure that she might be happily awake in the car seat for as much as an hour—but not much more. If you leave an hour before naptime, she'll be awake for an hour, and fall asleep, if you're lucky, for two hours. Then stop to feed her, change her, maybe eat dinner yourself, and get her back in the car for another hour awake and hope that brings you to your destination.

♡ Take Care of You: Travel by Night?

Some families drive at night so that baby sleeps through the trip. The car is quiet and traffic is light. Take into consideration your own sleep needs before doing this; a sleep-deprived parent at the wheel at 2:00 A.M. is a dangerous idea. Even if you're confident in your night-driving abilities, consider how tired you may be the next day. What might be good for baby could be terrible for you.

On an extended road trip, try to plan the route so that you can stop at parks or playgrounds along the way. Spread a blanket out on the grass in the shade of a tree and eat a picnic lunch while she watches other children playing on the jungle gym or ants climbing up the tree trunk. For older babies, a crawl or toddle in the sandbox for half an hour might be just what they need. If possible, break the trip up into shorter segments. Drive over two half-days instead of one long haul, perhaps visiting friends or family along the way.

If your baby is hungry and you're breastfeeding, don't remove her from her car seat while the car is in motion. Stop to nurse. (Some moms report leaning over baby's car seat to breastfeed from the adjoining seat without unstrapping their own seatbelt, but this can be tricky, not to mention hard on your body.)

Smart Mama Tricks: Pump on the Road

If you use a breast pump at home and your baby takes a bottle, consider bringing a portable unit (some plug right into the car) and expressing a bottle to feed the baby on the go. This, of course, assumes that someone else is doing the driving.

Traveling by Plane

There is nothing that instills panic in the minds of parents—as well as other passengers and flight attendants—as the thought of a baby's first airplane trip. Your baby may scream for hours, throw up all over you, and leak through her last dry set of clothes. Or your baby may sleep the whole way and wake only as the plane is coming in for a landing. You never know until you try. Now more than ever, remember your New Mama Mottos: Be prepared, be flexible, trust your instincts, and know that this plane ride, too, will pass.

The Not-So-Friendly Skies?

While traveling with an infant may be rough on parents, it isn't, under normal circumstances, hazardous to a healthy baby. There is no clear medical reason to forgo air travel until an infant is a certain age, although some airlines have restrictions on travel for infants only a few days old. Unless a trip is critical, you might consider holding off until your baby is more than two months old; airplanes tend to be germ-rich places, and when a baby under two months old gets a fever for any reason, it is a concern.

To some extent, whether you spend your flight reading a novel or passing out earplugs is a matter of your baby's temperament and luck. But you can tilt the odds.

♡ Take Care of You: Alternative Airports

When booking your flight, don't discount your small, local airport. Although it may be cheaper to fly from a major international airport, by flying from a smaller one, you may save your sanity by cutting down on drive time, while avoiding parking-lot shuttles and hour-long security lines.

Scheduling

When you make your reservations, think about your child's disposition at different times of the day. If she fusses every evening and needs to be walked for hours, a late-day flight is probably not a good idea. If she typically falls asleep easily and sleeps all night, maybe you're a candidate for a red-eye. (This is a risky move, though; fellow passengers who will grin and bear it when a baby is crying on a daytime flight can get downright nasty when their sleep is interrupted by a crying baby.) Know that sometimes babies are so excited by the newness of plane travel that, even though it's their normal bedtime, they will refuse to go to sleep and wind up overtired and fussy.

Have a Seat!

Consider purchasing a seat for your baby. Yes, she can fly free usually up to the age of two (or, on international flights, for a small fee), and the extra cost may be prohibitive, but having a guaranteed spot for your baby's car seat can make the difference between a merely stressful flight and torture. (You can put her down if she falls asleep, for one, and be able to lower your tray table and eat something yourself.) It's also a lot safer. Ask—it probably won't cost as much as your ticket and many carriers have greatly reduced fares for children under two.

♡ Take Care of You: Be Assertive

Don't be afraid to make a stink if you need help and you are not getting it. A tired mom with one or more fussy babies in tow, luggage to drag through the airport, and a quick connection to make, deserves help. The squeaky wheel does get the oil, and if you are overwhelmed, don't be shy; ask for assistance from the airline employees. If one person won't help you, ask to speak to a supervisor.

If you do purchase a seat, make sure to reserve the window for your baby; you won't be allowed to use the car seat in any other seat as it may block access to the aisle. You can also request a baby meal. Most airlines offer this option, which is usually a few jars of baby food.

♡ Take Care of You: Breastfeeding Privacy

If you're uncomfortable nursing in public, know that the high-backed seats of a commercial airliner give you a fairly private setting. In this case, ask for a window seat near the middle of the plane, with your traveling companion seated next to you. Most passenger foot travel is headed toward the bathrooms at the front and back of larger aircraft, so passersby will be kept to a minimum.

If you aren't purchasing an extra seat and are traveling with another adult or child, ask for an aisle and a window seat when you make your reservations. If you're lucky, the center seat will remain unoccupied. If not, whoever is assigned that seat will be happy to switch for your aisle or window and may, if your baby starts fussing before takeoff, look for a seat far away. (Hint: Boarding is not the time to worry about quieting your baby if you want to clear your row.) You may have been advised to ask for a bulkhead row. This tip makes sense, but you can't always get it; some airlines award bulkhead seats to good customers, not families with kids. Those that do hold bulkhead seats for families usually give them to travelers with babies before families of older children. And oftentimes these bulkhead seats have bassinets that fit into the tray table or sit on the floor.

Consider a seat in the front third of the airplane. Some airplanes have been remodeled to give front passengers extra leg room, and those few inches may make the difference between whether you can wriggle down to pick up a dropped rattle or not. If the front third is booked, try for one of the last few rows. You'll be close to the bathroom and at least have some floor space to pace with your baby.

Air Travel Tips

Here are some extra travel tips for travelin' babies and their mommies:

- When passing through security, wear slip-on shoes and keep ID and boarding pass in a pocket in your clothes. Your stroller, car seat, front pack or sling, shoes, and bags go through the x-ray machine at most airports, so you'll need to break everything down and then carry baby through the security gate barefoot, without losing your ID or stressing out about the impatient passengers in line behind you. No extra stuff at this point—cup of coffee, open food, and the like. You'll need both hands, one to hold the baby and one to gather your things at the other side.

- Gate-check your stroller, if you're using one. Tell the person checking boarding passes that you want a gate-check; he'll give you a special tag. Then you can push your baby all the way down the boarding ramp and unload your stroller just outside the door to the airplane. Put on the tag and leave the stroller there. It will be returned to you as you leave the airplane at your destination and it will be a lot easier to get your baby and her gear to the baggage area. (Occasionally, carriers do not offer this service. Check with your airline ahead of time.)

Smart Mama Tricks: Keep Lovey Close

Make sure you pack your baby's lovey or any other irreplaceable attachment item in your carry-on bag. You'll avoid potential meltdowns if your luggage is delayed or lost.

- Bring a car seat aboard. (Make sure that it's no wider than fifteen inches—that means it will fit in most coach seats.) You may also have to prove that your car seat is FAA-approved; if it doesn't say so on the label, it may in the instruction manual. Some infant seats will fit in the overhead compartment; if yours does, and you don't have a seat reserved for your baby, stash it there as soon as you get it on the plane. You can get it down later if it turns out you have an extra seat. If it doesn't fit, and the plane is full, you'll have to ask the flight attendant to check it for you. If you are using a convertible car seat (the kind that can be strapped in the rear-facing position for infants and switched to front-facing for older children), you may have to strap it in the front-facing position to fit it on the airplane. This isn't ideal, but it's safer than holding baby on your lap.
- Bring plenty of extra formula if you are bottle-feeding. Plane travel is dehydrating, and sucking will help protect your baby's ears from

pressure problems. If you're using powdered formula, bring plenty of water so you'll have it when you need it.

- Pack plenty of light cotton baby blankets. You'll use them to line the airplane bassinet, the changing table in the restroom, your lap in case of blowouts, and they'll serve as protection from the air conditioning and from bright lights overhead when your baby sleeps.

Smart Mama Tricks

Try to think of everything you might need before you stow your bags in the overhead bin. Grab those extra diapers, wipes, and blankets and keep them nearby. You don't want to spend the whole flight getting up and down for supplies.

- Pre-boarding. It's easier to get yourself and your gear stowed, strapped in, and settled before hordes of anxious passengers are trying to cram past you. (But if your baby is fussing and/or doesn't like to sit still for long, pre-board your partner with the carry-ons while you walk baby around at the boarding gate until the last possible minute—unless, of course, you are trying to clear your row.) Unfortunately, this courtesy is no longer offered on all flights. If there isn't an announcement for your particular flight, ask if you can pre-board; some airlines will respond to individual requests. If you're traveling as a solo parent with a baby, beg. Groveling is better than being trampled by impatient passengers as you are trying to stow your gear.

- Even if you always use a stroller, consider a front pack or other carrier for boarding and de-planing. You'll need your hands free while inside the plane to compile and carry all of your gear; and your stroller is *outside* the airplane.

- Nurse or bottle-feed your baby during takeoff and landing. The sucking and swallowing helps prevent discomfort in her ears from the changes in air pressure. If she's sleeping during takeoff, let her sleep; but if she's sleeping during landing, wake her up, that's when the pressure problems are the worst. If she's not interested in eating, use an eyedropper to put drops of water, juice, or milk in her mouth. She'll swallow them, and the swallowing will clear her ears. (Screaming will clear her ears too, of course.)

- Drink plenty of fluids yourself. (Bring a sports water bottle and get it refilled; it's easier to manage while wrestling a baby than a plastic glass or soda can.) This is critical if you are nursing.

- Bring extra baby clothes. And since your baby is not the only one who is going to get messy if she throws up or has a diaper blow-out, keep a change of clothes for yourself (at least one clean shirt and bra) and plastic grocery bags (for the mess) in your carry-on.

- Bring a favorite toy or two. Be on the lookout for found toys, too. (The laminated card with the picture of emergency exits somehow fascinates babies; you can make puppets out of barf bags or play stacking games with paper cups from the bathroom.)

- Bring a package of disposable earplugs. If your baby's screaming is getting you a lot of nasty looks from nearby passengers, stand up and offer the ear plugs around. You'll at least get a laugh, which may win a few people over to your side.

While You're on the Plane

One fiction that you need to drop is the idea that the flight attendant is always your friend. She may have been your friend when you were traveling on business, carrying a jacket and a briefcase, and quietly sitting in your aisle seat tapping away on your computer. She is not always your friend when you are pacing the aisle, trying to calm your screaming baby while simultaneously dodging the drink cart. Sometimes, you'll get a wonderful flight attendant who has—or remembers what it is like to have—young children. If the flight isn't too crowded, the attendant may volunteer to hold your baby while you go to the bathroom. Other times, despite your pleading, you'll get someone who insists on serving alcoholic beverages to all of the adult passengers on the flight before bringing your thirsty child her cup of water. With flight attendants, it's the luck of the draw.

The "I Have a Life" Guide to Baby's 1ˢᵗ Year

♡ Take Care of You: **Germ Warfare**

If airplanes are germ cesspools, their lavatories are the vortex of germ activity, with many travelers using a single bathroom over a long period of time. Bring anti-bacterial hand cleaner and/or tons of baby wipes and use them after every trip to the john.

Diapers in the Sky

Finding a place to change a diaper on an airplane can be a challenge—and infants always seem to have blowouts on airplanes. If your plane does not have a fold-down changing table in one of the bathrooms, you may want to try changing her somewhere else. (And realize that the changing tables that do exist are tiny.) The bathrooms themselves have no counter space and the floors are typically wet and sticky.

If you have a row to yourself, you might consider changing your baby on your seats. Wait until the flight attendant is not looking, and smile apologetically to nearby passengers if it's a smelly diaper. Whisk it into the airsick bag as quickly as possible. Speed is crucial here.

If there is no changing table and you don't have a row to yourself, your best bet is to change your baby on the floor or in the galley at the back of the plane. Try to stay out of the path of anyone who might walk by, and put down a blanket or two before you spread out your changing pad (again, the floor is likely to be pretty yucky). Or you can punt on the issue by slathering your baby's bottom with diaper cream and putting a super-absorbent diaper or double-diapers on her just before boarding and hope she doesn't poop before landing.

If you're switching planes as a solo parent and can't figure out how you are going to race with your baby, car seat, and diaper bag from gate to gate, try calling the airline. You may be able to arrange for help in the form of a chauffeured electric cart.

International Baby

If you're planning to travel internationally, give yourself plenty of time to get a passport for your baby. Getting a passport photo for an infant can be tricky. The instant cameras used for passport photos in photo shops don't work well with babies because they are designed to focus best at a distance of about four feet, and getting an infant's head to fill the photo requires getting in closer. Some photographers won't even try to produce passport photos of children under two. If you want to try the photo shop, bring a white blanket and an infant seat. The passport agency does not want your face in there with your baby's, and the photographer will have a better chance of getting a usable shot if your baby is comfortable, rather than being held in your hands at an awkward distance from your body.

Say Cheese!

You don't actually have to use an official passport photo. The shot needs to be taken head on, and your baby's eyes should be open. The background should be white or very light. You need two identical photos that are at least two inches square; the face, from the top of the head to the bottom of the chin, should measure between 1 and $1^3/_8$ inches.

So get out your ruler and scissors and start measuring photos. If you bought photos from the hospital photographer, try the wallet-sized prints—with some judicious trimming, these very well may work. Otherwise, lay your baby on a white blanket and stand over her (you may want to use a stool), taking shots from varying distances in hopes that one will be the right size.

In addition to your passports, bring a copy of your baby's birth certificate and your marriage certificate; they may come in handy. Some countries require immunization records, as well, so do your homework. If you are traveling without your spouse, bring a letter from him giving you permission to take your baby out of the country, and have a phone number where he can be contacted.

 Smart Mama Tricks: **Everything but the Kitchen Sink**

When traveling internationally, bring everything you need. Simple things such as diapers, diaper-rash cream, wipes, and formula are different in other countries and might not work well for your baby. Make sure you pack any baby medicines with you, as well, and if they are prescription meds, bring a copy of the doctor's prescription.

If you have the option, pick a foreign airline. They tend to be more baby-friendly than U.S.-based airlines.

International flights often accommodate bassinets—special little beds that go on the floor or attach to a bulkhead. Reserve one ahead of time; they are usually free of charge, but may be in limited supply.

If you are packing baby formula, make sure it is unopened. (Pack formula for the plane ride separately.) Otherwise, you may not be able to bring it into the country. Be sure to declare it, if asked.

Changing Time Zones

Crossing time zones can wreak havoc with a baby's schedule, but it doesn't need to result in a hungry, fussy baby. If you have an older baby who eats solid food, this is a good time to throw out your ideas of regular meal schedules. (And if you're nursing or bottle feeding, continue to offer on demand.) Babies are natural grazers because of their tiny tummies, and offering frequent small snacks can be an ideal way to help your child adjust to a new time zone.

Hotel Hints

When making your hotel reservations, it pays to ask for as much as possible in advance. Tell them you are traveling with a baby. Ask for a crib, a child-proofed room, a refrigerator, a room on the ground floor, whatever you need. When you do arrive, if the room does not suit your needs, ask to see another. Give yourself permission to be "high maintenance."

Smart Mama Tricks: Babyproof Your Room

Always check your hotel room for potential hazards. Get down on the floor at a crawling baby's eye level and block access to or remove electrical cords, cover electrical outlets, look through drawers, remove or block access to furniture that is easily tipped over, and knot Venetian blind cords out of reach, for starters. Even if the hotel personnel said that they babyproofed, see for yourself whether it was done correctly.

Your needs are greater than they were pre-baby, and you want to enjoy your vacation as much as possible.

Baby Equipment Rentals

Baby-gear rental businesses are sprouting up in many cities and popular vacation destinations. These companies provide all kinds of baby equipment for daily or weekly fees, including cribs with bedding, highchairs, car seats, strollers, beach toys, and CDs. Search online to see if your destination is covered by such a company and save yourself the trouble of packing so much stuff.

The Great Outdoors

Feeling adventurous? Plenty of families camp with babies. Again, it's a bit more work than it was during your pre-child days, but camping is "work" anyway. You still have to set up your equipment, cook your meals, etc. Now you're just doing your usual camping chores, plus taking care of your baby.

Fun with Dirt

Kids love dirt. Dirt loves kids. Therefore, the most challenging time to take baby camping is when baby is in the crawling stage. At this point, even the most dirt-tolerant parents may be thinking, "Enough already!" Before the crawling stage, you can keep your infant relatively confined to a large blanket on the ground or in a playpen while you conduct your chores.

Once she's walking, well, then you're chasing her all over the place, but at least she's not horizontal in the dirt all of the time.

When you camp with an infant, you may have to pack a few more things than you're used to. Along with your regular camping gear, consider:

- A portable playpen (somewhere safe to put the baby while you're doing camp chores, such as cooking)
- A waterproof crib pad for inside your sleeping bag, if you're sleeping with your baby (Remember to follow all of the co-sleeping safety rules.)
- A portable crib, if you're not
- A small inflatable wading pool for use as bathtub
- A large plastic bin to pack your clothes in and use as a baby bathtub
- Two extra-warm sleepers
- A large blanket for sitting on when you are outside the tent
- A highchair if your baby is eating finger foods (it will give her a chance to get the food in her mouth before it gets covered with dirt and can be used to contain her when you don't want to worry about her crawling into the fire)
- A front pack or backpack and/or a jogging stroller for hikes

Check out your campsite completely before letting your baby loose, in case previous campers left things behind that you don't want your baby to put in her mouth. Pay particular attention around campfires (whether lit or not; coals stay hot for a long time), cooking stoves, and bodies of water. Let the fun begin!

Chapter 13

From Bottles to Breast Pumps

If you've been nursing your baby at all, way to go! You've given your baby a loving, healthy start. If you're going to bottle feed now, you need to make a few informed decisions. Are you going to continue with breastmilk or switch to formula, or use both? If you choose to add formula to your routine, how does that work? And then there are breast pumps, bottles, and nipples to consider.

Express Yourself

Madonna did it. So did Celine Dion, Cindy Crawford, Anita Baker, Andie MacDowell, Demi Moore, Faith Hill, Goldie Hawn, Lisa Kudrow, and Heather Locklear. They were all nursing moms who breastfed and expressed milk for their babies. Whether you're returning to work, relieving engorgement, or pumping milk so you can have a night out, at some point most nursing mothers need to learn the art of expression.

However, if you don't have a reason to pump—for instance, no plan to go back to work or to attend an event to which you can't bring your baby—and you don't want to, then don't. Just plan on bringing your baby with you whenever you go out for more than a few hours until she's eating solids.

Pump It Up!

A breast pump is not as effective in removing milk from your breasts as your baby is, so it's important to establish a consistent routine to maintain your supply. The more frequently you pump, the stronger your supply, the same way frequent nursing works with your baby.

If you are returning to work, begin to express your milk about two weeks prior. This will help increase your production and get you into a pumping routine. You'll want to express about the same time as your baby would naturally nurse each day, or about every two to three hours in a twenty-four-hour period.

♡ Take Care of You: Pain-Free Pumping

Pumping your breasts should not hurt. If it hurts, stop and ask for help from your lactation consultant or the company that made the pump. Re-read the instructions and see if you can dial down the degree of suction on the pump to a level that is more comfortable for you.

Begin pumping for fifteen minutes using a double pump, or thirty minutes using a single pump (fifteen minutes on each side).

You might express very little milk your first few tries. It takes a while for your body to get used to this artificial suction device. It also takes time for your milk to let down. Eventually, you'll notice steady streams and bona fide long-distance sprays from your nipples, but for now, don't worry.

Any milk you express is important for your baby's growth. After about a week, you might be able to pump twenty-five ounces or more per day.

Smart Mama Tricks: One for the Bottle, One for the Baby

Milk flows best when you're relaxed. If you have difficulty with let-down when you pump, nurse your baby on one breast while pumping the other. Once your baby engages your milk ejection reflex, your milk will flow more freely.

Pick Your Pump

If you intend to express your milk on a regular basis, you'll need a breast pump that meets your individual needs. Keep your ultimate goal (whatever it may be) in mind while you shop, and consult your doctor or lactation consultant.

- How often will you use a pump: daily, weekly, or as needed? Are you returning to work or just planning to express an occasional bottle for date night?
- What can you afford? Is this an investment that you intend to use again with other babies or would it be more economical for you to rent?
- Will you be transporting your breast pump to work? Will you need a cooler or carrying case to transport milk back home?

- Will you be expressing in your car?
- What are your power resources?
- How much time do you have to express your milk?
- What kinds of accessories will you need?

 Smart Mama Tricks: **Don't Cook the Milk**

Even when stored at room temperature, fresh milk doesn't need to be heated. Boiling causes breastmilk to lose its precious immunity-enhancing properties. Even a slight warm-up in the microwave can hurt the milk and possibly harm your baby—microwave heat causes hot spots in a bottle that will scald baby's mouth. If you refrigerate your milk, you can heat it by holding the bottle under warm tap water or letting it stand in a bowl of warm water.

When choosing a pump, select the one that most closely imitates your baby's suckling pattern. Pumps that offer the most cycling per minute are the best. Look for pumps that offer thirty-four to fifty cycles per minute. That timing is most like your baby's nursing pattern. You also want a pump with adjustable suction rates.

With breast pumps, you truly get what you pay for. Better pumps will cost more, but they express more milk in a shorter period of time, are more comfortable to use, and are less likely to cause tissue damage.

You can contact your local WIC office, a lactation consultant or breast-feeding educator, or your local birthing center for additional information and recommendations.

You can also call or go to the Web sites of the following companies:

Medela: 800-835-5968, *www.Medela.com*
Hollister/Ameda/Egnell: 800-3234060, *www.Hollister.com*

Types of Breast Pumps

Try to choose a reputable brand like Medela or Hollister. These manufacturers have years of experience and a solid history behind their products. You wouldn't go to a seafood place if you wanted steak, so don't buy a breast pump from a company that specializes in something else.

> ♡ Take Care of You: **Get the Right Size**
>
> *Watch how your nipple enters and exits the flange. If your nipple is squashed, you might need a larger flange neck. Nipples should not rub or touch the sides. Contact the vendor you purchased your kit from to see about their return policy.*

Personal-Use (Portable) Electric Pumps

These pumps are durable and easy to transport, but often don't offer the optimum number of suction-release cycles. Portable electric pumps often come with accessory packages that offer cigarette-lighter adapters for use in your car. They have adjustable suction rates and allow you to double-pump. Prices vary, but plan on about $80 for a small single pump model to $200 to $300 for a fancier (and much more useful) double-pumper.

Hospital-Grade Pumps

These are simply the best and most efficient pumps around. Although they can be expensive to purchase (generally starting at around $800), most hospitals offer rental options for women who intend to pump frequently. Hospital-grade pumps come in several sizes and weights. Some are as light as four pounds while others weigh up to twenty pounds. The lightweight pumps are easily transported and come with adapters for automobile use.

Sometimes hospital-grade pumps are covered by insurance, particularly if your baby is premature or has a medical condition. Hospital-grade pumps are most effective and cost-efficient if you use them on a daily basis. Rental fees range from one to three dollars per day.

PUMP PROCESS (TWENTY TO THIRTY MINUTES)

1. Wash your hands with soap and water.
2. Wash all breast-pump equipment and assemble it according to the manufacturer's directions.
3. Find a comfortable location, just as you would to nurse your baby.

4. Gently massage your breasts or apply a warm washcloth.

5. Center the nipple in the plastic flange. If you are using an electric or battery-operated pump, turn it on the lowest/slowest setting first and increase the speed to match your baby's suck.

6a. Pump the first breast for about seven minutes. (If you are using a double pump, note that you'll follow the pump-massage-pump procedure without switching breasts.)

6b. Switch sides and pump the second breast for seven minutes.

7. Massage your breasts a second time.

8. Return to the first breast for five to seven minutes or until milk no longer flows, followed by the second breast for the same amount of time. Note: You might have to exchange containers midway through your expression session if your collection bottle becomes full.

9. When milk stops dripping, release suction at the breast as you would with your infant.

10. When you're finished, rub any excess milk off of your nipples and areola.

11. Pour the milk into a clean container for storage, or, if a lid is provided with your pump, screw it on tightly.

12 Label your milk with the date and the amount, and immediately refrigerate what you don't plan to use within eight to ten hours.

13 Detach the pump and disassemble any washable components. Clean everything according to the instructions in hot, soapy water. Air dry the components on a paper towel or a clean dishcloth.

Your Milk Store

Human milk can be stored at room temperature, refrigerated, or frozen. Each requires different handling and storage procedures.

If possible, it's best to use your breastmilk in the first few days after you've expressed it. Breastmilk is filled with living cells and delicate ingredients that are meant for your child immediately. Breastmilk loses many of its disease-fighting properties with freezing, with boiling, and over time. Although it's still the most perfect nutrition for your child, the near magical immunity properties of your milk are important, too. Temperature is the single most important factor in determining the length of time it's safe to store your milk.

Storage-Time Guidelines

Room Temperature	6–10 hours
Refrigerator	5–8 days
Freezer inside a Refrigerator	2 weeks
Self-Defrosting Freezer w/Separate Door	3–6 months
Deep Freeze at 0 Degrees	6–12 months

Defrosted or thawed milk can be stored for up to twenty-four hours in the refrigerator. If you don't have a refrigerator at your work site, you can refrigerate milk in an insulated cooler with ice packs until you get home or to the day care.

Discard any unused portion left in the bottle after your baby has eaten. It's hard to watch that liquid gold go down the drain, but bacteria from your baby's mouth make it unsafe for future feedings.

Smart Mama Tricks: **Keep It Cool**

Store your cooled or frozen milk in the back of your refrigerator or freezer. It's colder there, and your milk will be less affected by temperature changes from the frequent opening and closing of the door.

What about Bottles?

At some point, be it soon after the baby's birth, or some time later—say, when your favorite musician is on tour and you really, really want to go to a four-hour concert without worrying about what the loud music is doing to your baby's ears—it may occur to you that it would be nice if your infant had a friendly acquaintance with a bottle. You decide to introduce them.

Timing the Introduction

If you're breastfeeding and intend to occasionally use a bottle or eventually switch to a bottle full-time, timing is everything. Get her used to it when she is between four and eight weeks old. Too soon could affect your milk supply unless you pump regularly, too much later and she might not cooperate.

Once you start, conduct bottle practice every day. As soon as your baby has demonstrated that she is willing and able to suck from a bottle's nipple, you don't have to continue with daily bottles, but do remind her at least several times a week that milk does, indeed, also come in bottles.

Equipment Explained

The word "equipment" makes it sound like you are operating heavy machinery. It's not hard at all!

Bottles

First, there is the bottle. The three types of bottles (glass, plain plastic, and plastic with disposable liners) come in two sizes: small (four ounces) or large (eight or nine ounces).

That's where simplicity ends. Since each manufacturer tries to distinguish itself from the others, there are hordes of variations within each category. You will find short, fat bottles and long, thin ones. There are ones with a bend in the middle and ones with handles.

The general idea behind all these bottle designs is to make it harder for air to get into the baby. The bottle you choose doesn't matter all that much.

Nipples

What does matter is nipple choice. Nipples differ in size, shape, and flexibility. You want a nipple that most resembles the human breast. If you're bottle-feeding from the get-go, your options are open—a generic "breast" nipple is fine. But if you are transitioning to bottle-feeding from breastfeeding, you need to be more selective. The nipple's shape should resemble yours. For example, if you have large breasts with fairly flat nipples, your baby may be uncomfortable drinking from a long nipple on a small base. You may need to let your baby test a couple of shapes before you discover what works best.

According to the manufacturers' labels, the small, slow-flow holes are for newborns, while larger, faster-flow nipples are intended for older babies. But the manufacturer doesn't always know best—your baby may have a different idea. For instance, babies of mothers with strong let-down are used to gulping milk, and slow-flowing infant nipples may make them scream in frustration.

Even if you have the right nipple, you may not always get the right flow of milk, or even the same flow you got the last time. Turn the bottle upside down and shake it a few times. You should see a spritz of milk followed by slow, steady drops. You can adjust the flow by loosening or tightening the bottle's ring. You also may find that some supposedly "fast-flowing" nipples are slower than those advertised as "slow-flowing"—check the flow rates for yourself.

On the Menu

Next is the question of what goes in the bottle. If you're pumping and have a supply of breastmilk, you're all set. If not, you need to select a formula.

Which Formula?

There are milk-based and soy-based formulas. If your baby is normal birthweight and healthy, and if you have no reason to suspect food allergies, a regular formula based on modified cows' milk is usually the right choice. If your baby is extremely fussy, gassy, or spits up often, talk to your doctor about the possibility of food allergies or a sensitivity to cows'-milk protein. If your doctor thinks cows'-milk sensitivity is the problem, she'll probably tell you to switch to a soy-based formula. If you're a vegetarian or need to keep kosher, a soy-based formula is the next best thing to breastmilk.

There are also formulas that are specially processed to break down the milk proteins, which makes them easier to digest and less likely to cause allergies. These "protein hydrolysate formulas" taste terrible and cost twice as much as standard formulas, but can be a boon for some babies.

Formulas come packaged as a powder, concentrated liquid, or ready-to-serve liquid.

- For economy, availability, and shelf life, choose powdered formula mix. It is slightly more difficult to blend than the concentrated liquid, and you'll need safe water for mixing outside of the house.
- Concentrated liquid is a middle ground with simple mixing and a cost right in between. It doesn't work as well out of the house, because open cans need to be refrigerated and again you'll need safe water.
- Ready-to-feed is the Rolls Royce of formulas. Used exclusively, it can easily cost you a dollar per day more than powder. But ready-to-feed formula is unmatched among formulas for traveling convenience.

1. Boil the nipples and other bottle parts before the first use (this both sterilizes them and gets rid of the plastic flavor). After that, for a healthy, full-term infant you don't really have to sterilize them again as long as you have a chlorinated water supply. (Well water can be a concern. Have your water tested for safety or put the bottles in a pot and boil them for five minutes prior to each use.) For all subsequent washings, a run through the dishwasher (top rack) or hand washing in hot, soapy water will get them sufficiently clean.

2. Wash your hands, wipe off the top of the formula can, and mix the formula exactly according to the directions. Too little water can cause dehydration and too much water means your baby won't be getting enough calories.

3. Pour the formula into the bottle. Unless your baby is used to a warm bottle, she probably won't care if you serve it to her at room temperature or out of the refrigerator, although she may get used to (and come to prefer) the bottle temperature she gets most often.

DINNER IS SERVED: TIPS FOR BOTTLE-FEEDING

- First, get comfortable. Find a place where you can easily support the baby for a length of time without straining yourself. A comfy chair is a good choice.

- Second, tilt the bottle so the nipple is full of formula or breastmilk. Otherwise your baby will swallow excessive amounts of air during feeding. More air equals more spitup.

From Bottles to Breast Pumps

- Third, tilt your baby so that her head is higher than her stomach—she should be sitting up or reclining slightly. Never feed your baby when she is lying down. She can get ear infections. The eustachian tubes connect your baby's mouth and inner ear. When she drinks lying back, fluids run into her inner ear and stay there.
- Fourth, cuddle your baby. Hold her as if you were breastfeeding. This is especially true for newborns.

Smart Mama Tricks: No Bottle Propping

Never prop a bottle for your baby, as it could cause choking. If your baby cannot hold her own bottle, then someone else must hold the bottle for the baby. The flow of liquid does not stop even if the baby quits sucking on the bottle. A young baby cannot remove the bottle to protect her airway.

As your baby becomes able to grasp the bottle and take control, let her. Her coordination might be lacking at first. Sometimes babies frustrate themselves by knocking the bottle out of their own mouths. At those times, hold the bottle but let her grasp and tug it around. Before long, she'll be an old pro.

Chapter 14

Back to Work

The stay-at-home mom versus the working mom debate rages on. There are strong advocates on both sides, and the simple truth is you must do what's best for you and your family. Do you prefer the job of taking care of your own children full time, a career outside the home, or a combination of both? It's an individual choice, and no one can tell you what you should or should not do. There's so much to consider, such as whether you truly enjoy your career and want to work, whether you can or cannot bear to leave your baby in the care of someone else, and whether you can live on one income or must have two.

Money Matters

Most moms believe they must work out of financial necessity. If money is the primary issue in your decision, consider this: Many women have found that staying home with their child is less of a financial sacrifice than they feared. Sometimes, families' second incomes are far less profitable than they think. You see the figure on your paycheck but don't always fully consider how much is spent in related costs.

One study by the U.S. Department of Labor found that about 80 percent of a working mother's income is absorbed by job-related expenses. So if you earn $25,000 annually, your actual take-home pay might be valued around $5,000. That's just over $400 per month. It's not even unusual for couples to discover that their second income is entirely consumed by work-related expenses.

> ## ♡ Take Care of You: Listen to Your Own Heart
>
> *Sooner or later, whether you stay at home or go back to work, those on the other side of the fence will try to guilt you into thinking you've made a bad decision. Don't get sucked into an argument that simply comes down to individual choice. Stay the course and continue to do what works best for you and your family.*

You Do the Math

Consider some of these factors when making your decision.

Career paths. Many women have invested a great deal of time and effort into their careers and enjoy working too much to consider staying home. You might decide that an interruption would compromise your career goals.

Clothing and transportation expenses. The cost of commuting can be substantial whether you drive, take the bus, or carpool. For some urban families, one vehicle would be enough if not for the second job. Car payments, tolls, parking, gas, and service all add up. Then there's also the cost of maintaining a professional wardrobe—business clothes, shoes, and dry cleaning.

Cost of childcare. Daycare can be expensive. Expect to pay at least $700 to $1,200 per month for infant care, depending on where you live and what type you choose. If you have more than one small child, expenses could double.

Food expenses at work versus home. Unless you're the kind of person who packs an inexpensive sack lunch every day, workday food expenses can put a dent in your pocketbook. The average homemade lunch costs less than $1. The cheapest fast-food meal is more than four times that. That's around $800 per year minimum, not counting trips to the vending machine for snacks. The other, often hidden, food expense to consider is the cost of ordering out at night because everyone is too tired or impatient to prepare a meal.

Health insurance. Babies get sick from time to time, and health insurance is an essential benefit most employers offer. Well-child visits during the first three years of life will outnumber those needed for the ten years following. A trip to the doctor's office can easily set you back $150 or more, depending on what treatment is medically indicated. Most insurance companies offer copays for as little as $10 per visit.

Intellectual stimulation and camaraderie. Staying at home can be isolating and even boring at times. Your baby is always happy to interact with you, but sometimes you'll miss adult conversation and the friendly camaraderie of your fellow employees. Many stay-at-home parents start playgroups, write newsletters, take up hobbies, and volunteer at schools to combat feelings of isolation.

Self-esteem and social status. Many people define themselves in terms of what they do. Losing that role can leave some parents feeling depressed or socially diminished. There's a real lack of appreciation in the world for the hard work, skill, and ingenuity of stay-at-home parents. Making the transition from corporate ladder climber with power lunches, to diaper changer with playdate picnics can cause a real identity crisis.

Taxes from a second income. First, take into account all of the taxes deducted from your paycheck to calculate its true take-home value. Then, if your second income raises the family into a higher tax bracket, then you have to figure the extra taxes paid on the primary income as expenses related to your secondary income. In plain English, if your income puts the family into a 22 percent tax bracket when it would otherwise be in an 18 percent bracket, the extra 4 percent taken out of your partner's check is an expense related to your employment.

Time. Time is money, so they say. Much of the expense of the dual-income lifestyle originates in lost time. You don't have time to paint the living room, so you hire a painter. You don't have time to cook, so you order out. You don't have time to shop for the best prices, so you buy whatever you can get quickly. Moderately careful stay-at-home parents can sometimes save more than they would earn at a regular job simply by investing their time wisely.

If, after you consider all the factors involved, you find that your job is less profitable than you thought, maybe you can consider becoming a full-time parent for a while. Conversely, you may find that your income is high and decide that it's needed to maintain your current living standards.

Job-Related Expenses Worksheet

Taxes $_____
    (Taken from your check and possibly your partner's)

Work Clothing $_____
    (Purchase price, dry cleaning)

Transportation $_____

    (Car payment, parking, fuel, insurance)

Eating Out/Snacks $_____
    (List only the difference over home cooking.)

Daycare $_____

Office Gifts $_____
    (Birthdays, funeral flowers, etc.)

Convenience Services $_____
    (Things you could do if you had time)

Total Expenses: $_____

Gross Income: $_____

Value of Your Job (Income – Expenses): $_____

When and How

Returning to work should be a gradual process. Talk to your employer before you start maternity leave. Discuss the possibility of returning at part-time status or for half days for the first few weeks back. Ask if you can return on a Thursday or Friday, creating a long transitional weekend to get mentally prepared and back on track. Other options to consider include job sharing, working from home, or flexible scheduling. Some small, progressive businesses might even allow your young, non-mobile infant to come to work with you.

How Long to Stay Home

How long you are able to stay home before returning to work will depend on many things, including how long you have for maternity leave and how long you want to stay home. This can be a tough decision. How you felt during pregnancy is often different from how you feel once your baby is born. You may be able to negotiate a period of twelve weeks, per the Federal law on family leave, called the Family Medical Leave Act (FMLA).

♡ Take Care of You: **Set Limits While on Leave**

Avoid the temptation to be available to answer work calls when you're home with your baby on leave. Once people at work know you'll answer the phone or e-mail, it may be difficult to get a moment's peace. Keep in contact with work while on maternity leave, but make sure it's on your own terms.

Remember, go back when you are ready to, but at the same time be reasonable. The best thing you can do is get yourself and your baby used to the working routine if you do plan on returning.

Pump It Up at Work

There are probably few things as generally unpleasant as sitting in a toilet stall at work over your lunch break, pumping milk for your baby. That's dedication. Fortunately, things are changing for breastfeeding moms on the job all over the country. Employers are being educated on how maintaining a breastfeeding-friendly workplace benefits everyone.

Using a breast pump at work shouldn't be problematic. There are many ways to pump discreetly and easily while at work. If you have your own office, that's ideal. Simply shut your door. If you have a lock, use it. Some mothers hang a sign on the door saying simply "Do Not Disturb"; others hang signs that proudly declare "Pumping in Progress."

If you don't have your own office, find a space that works for you (other than the bathroom stall, if you can help it). Some businesses actually provide rooms for pumping moms. Check with your employer to see if you can help set one up in your workplace.

If there's no pumping room available, perhaps there's a vacant office or meeting room you can use for short periods of time. Check for any available space. Also, be sure to get clearance from your supervisor to do this; you don't want an expectant group of coworkers banging down the door for a meeting while you're holed up inside pumping. Another alternative would be to pump at the daycare or other place your child is during the day. You may even be able to get a true feeding in.

Modern Conveniences

If being away from baby forty-plus hours a week seems like too much, seek a schedule that is more flexible for your current needs. Consider a part-time work situation, a combination of working at home and working in your office, or job sharing.

Telecommuting

If you can connect to the Internet and read e-mail from home, you may be able to work from home some of the time. If you have certain duties that you could manage from home, talk to your supervisor.

Working from Home

Working entirely from home can give you the best of both worlds—you're home with your baby and you're making money. It may sound ideal, but it can also have some bad points. There's a fine balance that has to be met to make a work-at-home arrangement not only pleasurable, but profitable, as well.

♡ Take Care of You: **Tax Breaks**

If you work from home, consult your tax consultant about tax deductions you can take for your home office and other related expenses.

Whether it be freelance work, in-home sales work, or something else, you first must find an opportunity that suits you. Keep your eyes and ears open for any job that fits your situation. You can find jobs doing anything from stuffing envelopes to making jewelry. Be very careful about jobs that ask you for money up front. Check out the business in detail. Ask to speak to employees. And remember, things that seem too good to be true often are.

♡ Take Care of You: Set Office Hours for Home

Having a home office is not as easy as it sounds. Sometimes you'll feel like work is calling to you, even though you'd rather be with your family. Having twenty-four-hour access to work can have that effect. Set "home office hours" and stick to them.

However, there are plenty of legitimate businesses that need help on a part-time basis, and many of these jobs can be done in your home. If you can't find a job you're looking for, take inventory of your skills. Is there a business you could run from home? A product or a service you could sell? Do you have a way to market your service or product? Can you conduct your business over the Internet?

Plenty of options exist, from Web-page or graphic design, to bookkeeping or accounting, to event planning or a home-party business.

Fitting a Home Job into Your Life

While taking care of your baby and your home and yourself, some-where in there, you have to find the time to do your job. Skip the tendency to put it off until bedtime. This will only make you sleep-deprived, cranky, and push your body out of whack. Instead, try to work out a childcare schedule with your partner, or hire a sitter the necessary daytime hours a week so that you can get the job done.

> ### ♡ Take Care of You: All Work and No Play...
>
> *Make sure you discuss childcare duties with your working spouse before taking an at-home job. You may need him to take over baby care the moment he gets home in the evening so that you can start in on your assignments. This can be grueling for both of you and for your relationship because no one gets a break. Factor in both parents' need for downtime before you take on the job.*

Job Sharing

What about sharing your job with someone else? New moms who are elementary school teachers often use this approach, teaching the same class on different days. Perhaps you each work two full days and alternate Fridays each week. Some jobs have you alternate three- and two-day weeks. Or you might be able to work five half-days.

Working 24/7

The hard part about being a working mom is that you're not done when you come home. You can't just sink into the couch and kick your feet up to the evening news like you used to. Your job as a mother is not nine to five—it continues around the clock. There's no way you can handle all your responsibilities without help. You and your partner must divvy up the household chores.

Think of everything that needs to be done to run your household. Make a list. You may wish to trade some chores back and forth. This works well for tasks that no one wants. You may divide by whatever jobs you each prefer if it's divided evenly enough and you and your partner are fine with it. Once you have done this, your house will run much more smoothly. You and your partner can quit arguing about dishes and get back to real life.

One of the most important skills you can learn is how to say no. "No" doesn't mean "never." It simply means "not right now." You have a lot on your plate. There will be time in the future for you to take on projects, volunteer, and do other things. The first year should be about your family.

Separation Anxiety

You've just spent every minute of your life with your new baby, and now the focus is changing. In addition to getting back into the swing of things at work, you also have the challenge of separation from your new baby. It is perfectly normal to miss your baby when you first go back to work.

Yours

There are a few things you can do to help ease the pain of being apart.

- Ensure you've got the best childcare available. A little apprehension is natural, but if you are sincerely worried about your baby's well-being while you're away, you're not going to get much work done.
- Consider visiting your child or having your partner visit your child during the day to help ease your fears. If you hire someone to care for your baby at your home, try to go home for your lunch break.
- Place photos of your baby on your desk or your locker—somewhere you'll see them. The frequent sight of your baby's face may help you transition into days of separation.

Your Baby's

Some infants can be blissfully unaware that their parents have gone to work during the day. They are aware of their new surroundings and the people around them, but it might not be distressing to them. What may be distressing to your infant is a sudden change in lifestyle.

Did you pick a childcare facility that will listen to what your baby's schedule has been? Do they have enough people or few enough babies to give your infant the attention he needs? Are there consistent caregivers that he can get to know and bond with? (See Chapter 16, Mind the Baby, for more information on childcare.) As long as your infant has his needs met by regular people whom he has come to know, he should not become overly stressed about being someplace other than with you. However, as your baby gets older, separation anxiety can become a big issue. This can happen as early as about five or six months. It can also happen later. Or you may get lucky and your baby will skip it altogether.

Stay-at-Home Dads

More and more fathers are moving away from employment outside the home to full-time fathering and housekeeping. It's an arrangement that benefits the entire family. Mothers can continue on their career paths uninterrupted, knowing that their children are being cared for by someone who loves them. Fathers can enjoy the special parent-child relationship that usually belongs to Mom.

Consider these factors:

- Who has more earning potential?
- Who has more job-growth opportunity?
- Who has the better, less costly insurance?
- Who is better suited to staying home?
- Who wants to stay home?

Couples considering this move need to consider all the financial factors listed earlier, but pay special attention to the social and emotional criteria. There aren't very many traditional role models for stay-at-home fathers. Studies show that the isolation of staying home and the loss of self-esteem and status from leaving their jobs hits men harder than it hits women. The support groups that exist for moms are not always as open to dads—and sometimes it takes Dad some time to get used to hanging out with groups of womenfolk.

However, organized dad's groups are starting up all over the country. Check out *www.slowlane.com* for valuable information and resources for the stay-at-home dad.

The Best of Both Worlds

Is it possible to secure the corner office and still have a great family life? Can you be a working mother and still have a child who knows who you are? The answer is absolutely yes; you just have to work hard at it. And remember, things will never be perfect. The key to success is isolating trouble spots and working to improve them, while always appreciating the good things you do have.

Chapter 15

Full-Time Mama

The decision to stay home is not an easy one. You may be worried about losing your career or your mind. Perhaps you're worried about finances. You may have decided long before you ever became pregnant that home was where you wanted to be once you had children. Or you may have been positive that you would return to work—all the way up until the moment you held your newborn in your arms, at which point your mind inexplicably and irrevocably changed. Your choice of becoming full-time caregiver to your baby does not make you old-fashioned, conservative, or any of the other labels that might be thrust upon you. You're simply a woman who knows what she wants.

The Toughest Job You'll Ever Love

What happens when you realize that your dream job isn't quite what you expected? Being a fabulous mother of three is an easy concept but a difficult task. Be cautious about forming exalted expectations for stay-at-home momhood.

Talk to other mothers and take in both the good and the bad. Ask them how their lives differ from what they'd anticipated. You'll hear some women complain about lack of sleep and others excitedly babble about their little one's latest accomplishment.

Smart Mama Tricks: Your Work Is Play

Your baby learns through playing. So all of the playing that you can do with your baby is not only fun time, but productive time. Sing learning songs, like your ABCs. Count out the number of objects you lay on a blanket or the number of kisses you give your baby. These are all learning situations for him and an valuable way to spend your day.

Ready (or Not)

With prior planning, you may come into the home-parenting situation more prepared to deal with its ups and downs. If you've had long-term plans, you're probably more financially prepared for the prospect of staying home. You may also be more emotionally ready for the task at hand. Of course, even if you have some trouble at first, this is not an indicator of failure. There's a learning curve involved, whether or not you had time to plan ahead.

The One-Income Family

You may think that living on one income is impossible in this day and age. Of course, it depends on each family's individual circumstances, but it is possible for many. You'll just have to make some changes in the way you live.

Even though your family will lose your paycheck, the truth is that you are also free of a few extra expenses. Sit down and think of all the things you'd no longer have to pay for if you didn't work: transportation, a professional wardrobe, daycare, and other hidden costs (see page 189 for a job-related expenses worksheet).

Think Before You Spend

There are many things that you can do to make the shift more economically feasible. By lightening your load, you can make it more possible to enjoy your new job as a stay-at-home mom.

First, reduce your spending. Can you consolidate your debt into one payment at a better rate? Can you refinance your home? Rates fluctuate, so sometimes you can get a better deal than when you first applied. Start planning menus to help save on grocery bills. Some stores actually have online grocery shopping. While you may spend $5 on the service, you eliminate all impulse buying and you don't have to go inside the store. But even if that doesn't work out, planning ahead can keep you from spending more than you wanted and keep you from heading to a restaurant on a whim.

Most important of all, try to get off the work-and-spend treadmill. American society is incredibly consumer-driven. We buy far more than we actually need. We compare ourselves—and our cars, our furniture, and our homes—endlessly with our neighbors and friends and family. Maybe you don't have to wear the latest fashions or upgrade to the newest computer (or even own more than one). Do you need that $100-plus-per-month cable TV subscription? Or could you subscribe to a $10-per-month DVD-by-mail service instead?

Accept hand-me-down baby clothes from friends. Infants grow so fast they don't have time to wear anything out. There are so many baby-gear items that aren't absolutely necessary, such as a changing table (you can place a changing pad on the bathroom counter or a dresser top), burping cloths (use old cloth diapers or dish towels), diaper-wipes warmer (if baby is used to room-temperature wipes or damp washcloths, she won't complain), and electric bottle warmers and bottle cleaners (if you want to warm a bottle, use a bowl of warm water; to clean the bottle, soap and water are fine), to name a few. When you're creative, you can cut corners and save money in so many ways.

♡ Take Care of You: Stay Focused

When you remember the reasons why you're staying home, it can make the execution of the plan easier for you. Let chores slide in favor of your baby. This little bundle of joy is the essence of your life, and no amount of work can overshadow that.

Identity Crisis

Your role as a stay-at-home mom is different from any other job you've had in your life. You don't really fit in with the working crowd, and you're new to the mommy crowd. It's awkward at first, but you'll get the hang of it.

Going from having a defined title at your job to being a stay-at-home mom is a tough transition. Suddenly you might be a housekeeper, caregiver, cook, chauffer, and banker. This is why you need to define your new role. (Supermom is not a title you want to even begin to try on, let alone earn.) Both you and your spouse must be on the same page when it comes to sharing responsibilities.

Divide and Conquer

Question: What can you reasonably accomplish during the day? Answer: A lot less than you think. Hello! You have a little baby. New moms inevitably try to take on too much. Do not expect to keep your baby entertained and safe while maintaining a spotless household, paying the bills, grocery shopping, and cooking dinner every night. Oh, and don't forget the laundry.

There will be many days where nothing seems to get done. Perhaps the baby has a cold and you spend the entire day breastfeeding and holding her. Or maybe you have a fussy baby that needs constant attention every day. That's okay. Everything else can wait. In this new life of yours, caring for your baby—without losing yourself—is the most important job you can do. You are laying the foundation of trust and love that will last a lifetime.

Talk with your partner about your expectations. If you don't discuss these issues, your life will quickly spin out of control. Your partner may expect one thing and get another. You'll be wondering why he's not helping, and he may not even know you expect help.

Play to likes and talents when divvying up chores. If he's a great chef, let him cook a couple of nights a week, while you supply the groceries for the meal and then clean up. Or if you absolutely hate garbage and he absolutely hates laundry, trade.

Just because you don't have an income doesn't mean you're not "working" all day long. When you partner comes home, he needs to keep up his fair share of the household duties. Keep talking, try not to accuse each other of slacking (when, in reality, you're both doing more and sleeping less than ever before), and seek a reasonable compromise.

Smart Mama Tricks: A Daily Shower?

From your earliest days home, try to shower at the same time every day, placing the baby safely in a bouncy seat or bassinet on the floor, next to the tub, where you can see her. Installing a clear, see-through shower curtain will help. Baby will come to know that at this time of day, she relaxes and listens to the lulling sounds of the water—and perhaps to your lovely singing voice, as well. (Given the acoustics, this would be an excellent time to serenade her.) You may just get a shower every day for the entire first year.

Save Your Sanity

In your new life as a stay-at-home mom, you may sometimes look around and realize that the only people you've talked to that day are under the age of one, *Sesame Street* has become your favorite show, and you're humming silly kids' songs in the shower. When you notice motherhood taking over your life, it's time to take a break.

Get Out of the House

The easiest way to stay sane? Grab your babe and go somewhere. Go out to the mall and walk around, or go to a park or library to read in peace while baby naps in the stroller or front pack. What do these activities have in common? The company of other people, of course. You can't just talk to your baby all day. You need to have adult conversations as well. So get out there and talk to people.

Hopefully, you've started to establish a circle of like-minded parents to hang out with. Remember the wisdom of creating a parenting village (see Chapter 10, "Your Parenting Village"). You need this now more than ever.

 Smart Mama Tricks: **Talk, Talk, Talk**

Your baby learns language through interaction with you. Months before he actually speaks to you, he is processing and learning your voice and your words. Describe out loud everything you do with him, from changing his diaper to looking for bugs in the dirt. Put everything into a running monologue—and look forward to the day when all of those words pour out of his mouth right back at you.

Try some organized activities for moms and babies. Mom-tot music classes, baby gym classes, and swimming classes abound. Perhaps you can find a mother's walking group or a playgroup for babies. There are many activities that you can find to do with other parents and babies. Getting out will also expose you to potential new friends.

When You Have to Stay In

There may be reasons you can't get out of the house, but this doesn't mean that you are destined to go nuts in your home. Sometimes it's a transportation issue. You might not have a car during the day and it's pouring rain. Or maybe your baby isn't feeling well. Perhaps you live far from town. No matter what the reason, don't panic. You can find ways to stay motivated at home, as well.

♡ Take Care of You: **It's Not All about Cooking and Cleaning**

Don't be put off by the thought of staying home just because you don't like doing dishes, laundry, and other housework. The main focus when you stay home should be caring for your family. Housework is a potential extra, but you'd be doing some even if you worked outside the home. This is about you and your baby.

Call a friend whom you haven't talked to in a while and gaze out the window as you chat. Watch a bit of television or a DVD. Catch up on the news or read a book you've kept waiting on the shelf. Surf the Internet. Do what it takes to stay rational and try to get out when you can.

Combat "Mommy Brain"

Keeping yourself intellectually stimulated is tough when you're a stay-at-home parent. Is there something you've always wanted to learn? A musical instrument? Watercolor painting? A foreign language? While you may not have attended a class in years, joining a casual class a couple of times a week might be just what you need to keep your brain cells firing. See if you can't find a sitter a couple of times a week or have your partner watch the baby while you take a day or night class or an online course.

Consider continuing or furthering your education or finishing a degree. Maybe you'd like to take a course in child development to help you in parenting (some of these classes allow babes-in-arms to attend). Take anything you'd be interested in, even if it doesn't seem that practical. What about a baking or a sign-language course? Perhaps you could join (or start) a book club.

This doesn't have to be an academic challenge. Many community centers offer classes on belly dancing, water aerobics, and other fitness specialties you may not have thought of. Regardless of what you choose, decide on a goal to motivate you. The point is to get out of the house and be with other adults for a while and enjoy yourself.

A Daily Plan

What are we going to do all day? It's often the first thing on a new mom's mind each morning. You might feel like you'll go crazy if you have nothing planned to pass the time. You may love a routine, but nowadays flexibility is a must. Find out what you like to do with your baby and plan for these activities.

Fill your calendar with fun and laughter, playdates and long walks in the park, and don't be afraid to go out and have adventures in the city, at the zoo, or at the museum. Just remember to alternate periods of play with periods of rest. You can overschedule even a small baby. And, of course, you need your rest as well.

♡ Take Care of You: You're Worth Every Penny

If you find yourself measuring your self-worth by the size of your paycheck, take heart: Salary.com recently valued the job of a stay-at-home mom (housekeeper, teacher, cook, driver, psychologist, etc.) in excess of $130,000 a year.

Chin Up

People out there might make rude comments to you about your choice to stay home. These small-minded people aren't able to see that raising children is the most important task we do, a task that is best left to those who are smart, competent, and committed. Anne Lamott said it best: "A hundred years from now? All new people." You are raising the next generation of world citizens. What could be more important than that?

Remember that your children are only young once and that the time will fly by; being with them as they grow is an investment in their future. Chances are you'd regret missing these important years of your child's life, but you'll never regret personally experiencing every exciting milestone.

Chapter 16

Mind the Baby

The first time you leave your baby with someone, anyone but you, is a big step—and typically that's simply entrusting her with your partner or another close family member for an hour or two. Leaving your baby in the hands of a paid childcare provider can be difficult indeed, whether it's for a forty-hour workweek or just so you can run errands for an hour. By exploring a wide variety of choices and options, rest assured that you can arrange childcare that works well for you and your family.

Know Your Options

In general, you will choose from among the following:

- **Family Care.** Your mother, your sister, your cousin, or another family member watches your child while you're away, either at their home or yours, paid or unpaid.
- **Babysitters.** These caregivers come to your home, and they range from the neighborhood teen to professional babysitting services.
- **Au Pairs.** An au pair is sometimes trained, sometimes not, usually in her late teens through her twenties, and often from a different country. She lives in your home and helps you with childcare for a set number of hours a week in exchange for a room of her own and a basic salary.

- **Nannies.** Nannies are generally more highly trained and experienced than au pairs and have chosen childcare as a lifelong profession. You may opt for a live-in nanny or a nanny who comes in daily to help you out.
- **Home Daycare.** These smaller daycare providers usually operate out of their home and care for approximately six children of varying ages.
- **Commercial Daycare.** This is the well-known type of licensed facility that houses numerous children, usually broken down into groups by age.

 Smart Mama Tricks: **Expand Your Horizons**

Don't confine your search to childcare centers near your home. That can drastically limit your choices. Also consider places near your workplace or your partner's workplace. You may find a perfectly good location at the halfway mark, so try not to restrict yourself too much geographically.

Before you make a decision, fully explore what is available around you. Ask your friends who have children what types of childcare options they know of in your area. Talk to the people you work with and those your partner works with. Check with childbirth educators in your area, as they often work with new families and may be aware of options.

The "I Have a Life" Guide to Baby's 1st Year

206

In-Home Care

In-home care means that a caregiver looks after your baby in his natural habitat, your home. This option can be expensive, like employing a live-in nanny. Employing a friend or family member may be more cost-effective.

ADVANTAGES OF IN-HOME CARE
- Your baby remains in familiar surroundings with all supplies needed for his care.
- Your baby receives consistency of care and full attention from one individual who will develop a relationship with him.
- Flexible hours may include evenings and weekends.
- Your baby is not exposed to illness from other children.
- Parents do not have to pack up little ones on cold mornings and transport them to daycare.
- If a parent must travel, in-home care can provide around-the-clock supervision.

DISADVANTAGES OF IN-HOME CARE
- It's difficult to monitor the quality of care your infant receives.
- It's hard to find someone outside of the family who can place the same investment in your child as you do.
- When your caregiver is sick, alternative care may be tough to find.
- It's a high-stress job and has high turnover rates (about 90 percent annually).

- It's expensive.
- It can be isolating, with little peer-group interaction for your growing baby.

Who's the Lucky Person?

You may be looking at in-home care in the form of a stranger, or in the form of a trusted family member. Either way, you want to be sure the person is right for the important job at hand.

Interviewing Candidates

When you're looking at outside candidates, you are dealing with an individual—a free agent, of sorts—and you need to ask different questions and do additional and thorough research. Ask all candidates for an in-home care position these questions to start with:

- What previous experience do you have with newborn care?
- What are the costs/fees involved?
- What special arrangements will you require (benefits, private room, evenings and weekends free)?
- Do you smoke, drink, or use drugs?
- Do you have transportation and a valid driver's license and are you insured?
- Do you have any health concerns that might interfere with the job?
- Can you work flexible hours?

- Are there other children (her own) in your care?
- Can you provide full-time care, if needed?
- Why did you leave your last job?
- Have you ever been charged with a crime?

Ask specific questions about her childcare philosophies, what she would do in different situations, for example when the baby won't stop crying or refuses to nap; see if her solutions mesh with yours. Ask for references and call them. Every one of them. Ask if they would hire this provider again. Were they pleased with the quality of care? Were there any concerns?

Listen to your intuition when making a final decision. If something just doesn't seem right, you can either interview again or find another provider. You want to make the best decision based on all available information.

All in the Family

You probably feel more comfortable using family for childcare because you know the people who are caring for your baby, and they presumably have a vested interest in your baby and genuine love for him, as well. In fact, a big advantage of using a family member for childcare is that family doesn't normally "disappear." This person that your baby bonds with and falls in love with will continue to be a part of his life long after he starts school and no longer needs full-time daycare.

For many families, this works out well. You typically pay your family members less (if at all) to help out while you work. They're often more flexible in terms of hours, particularly if they are retired. Your baby will be either in your home or in a relative's home that is familiar to him and to you.

This option usually results in fewer sick days, due to your baby's lack of exposure to other children. However, if the family caregiver is sick one day, you're left high and dry.

Good Families Gone Bad

What do you do when you arrive home from work to see your three-month-old spitting applesauce all over his face with Grandma holding the spoon? Or your infant crying by himself in her crib while Aunt Jane explains that he's simply exercising his lungs and if she picks him up she'll spoil him?

> ♥ Take Care of You: **A Contingency Plan**
>
> *Try to spare hurt feelings up front. In the beginning, sit down and have everyone involved agree that if it's not working out for either party, you'll agree to amicably part ways with no hard feelings. This is not a foolproof precaution, but it's worth a shot.*

When your philosophies in child rearing don't match, you don't have the control over a family member that you do over other providers. If the baby's grandmother disagrees with you about when to start solids, how to dress your baby, or other parenting decisions, you may find your wishes being violated while you're not at home.

And it can get worse. What do you do when the family member just doesn't work out? They're family, after all. It can't help but be personal. Terminating this arrangement can be awkward and hurtful for both of you. Whatever your reason or your family member's reason is for ending the agreement, be kind about it; you don't want to ruin relations with a well-loved relative over this.

Babysitters

Even if you don't need regular child care, you'll probably want a babysitter at some point. Or this person might help out a bit while you catch up on things at home. No matter why you might need supplemental child care, babysitters are indispensable.

Smart Mama Tricks: **Pay for Training**

If your community offers babysitting classes and your regular baby-sitter hasn't attended them, offer to pay for a course and give her a ride to the venue. You will profit from her added skills and confidence, and she becomes more marketable.

The Neighborhood Teen

Sometimes a local teenage girl is adequate when it comes to babysitting needs. You could also post a notice at your local college's child development or early childhood education department. Ask what the current going rate is in your community, and prepare yourself for the new babysitting wage. Your parents may have paid sitters $1 per hour when you were young. You're more likely to pay between $6 and $15 per hour, depending on where you live and whom you hire. The wage should match her experience and what she is responsible for during her stay.

A nice trick to use is to invite your new babysitter over to meet the baby before her first night. You can keep a low-profile and the two can get used to each other—with you in the next room in case something goes wrong.

Smart Mama Tricks: **Honorary Grandparents**

Don't discount older adults in your search for a caregiver. Oftentimes these folks delight in the fact they're actually getting paid to be a grandparent. They're usually experienced and unlikely to be distracted by talking to their boyfriends on their cell phone all day.

Another path is a babysitting service. The nice thing about a babysitting service is that they do all the screening for you. They also hunt down someone for whatever dates and times you may need. They may or may not take requests for certain providers.

Unlike the girl who lives in the neighborhood, these sitters drive themselves to your house and drive themselves home—always a blessing after an evening out. You'll probably pay a bit more for the service than you might pay your local teen. There are also usually a minimum number of hours that they will work, so if you don't stay out that long, you'll still have to pay for it. Sitters from a service are usually older and have more experience, but the drawback is that you might not have a chance to meet them until they show up at your door, ready to work.

Full-Time Help

If your finances permit, you might even consider hiring someone full-time to help you with your baby. This is especially helpful if you're a working mama, or if you have multiple children!

Au Pairs

Au pairs are great for many types of situations, including families with odd work hours, multiple children, or other special needs. Typically students or young people who love to travel, they usually come from au pair agencies located around the world. The amount of training and experience of each au pair varies greatly, as does the language your au pair speaks, depending both on the agency and the au pair.

Most au pairs are allowed to stay with a family for only a year or two. This can be heartbreaking to a young child when she has grown attached to her caregiver. Sadly, the rules are fairly inflexible. Keep this in mind when choosing an au pair as your form of child care. Developing babies thrive with a consistent caregiver, and broken attachments can have an emotional impact.

Most au pairs are supposed to speak English, though this doesn't always work out as well as some families hope. On the other hand, some families choose an au pair mainly for her ability to speak a different language to their baby. Be sure to screen not only your agency, but also the au pair, for your desired level of English-speaking ability.

Nannies

Nannies can be an expensive choice—but what price is too high for Mary Poppins? For some, the concept of a nanny may seem quaint and outdated, but this is still a popular option.

One of the biggest benefits of a nanny is that your child receives one-on-one care from the same person every day. This can be a huge advantage for some families, particularly if you have special requests or your child has special needs. Nannies can also stay longer-term than au pairs, even several years, avoiding painful breaks in emotional attachment.

Many nanny-training schools offer placement services. While this sounds good, it can also be quite costly. Some services charge over $1,000 to help you find a nanny. The good part is that they handle all the criminal and background investigations that may be difficult for you.

Other nannies simply have on-the-job training. They may have years of experience or could be just starting out, with only babysitting experience. Some are college students looking to have a steady income while finishing school in the evenings, while others intend to make childcare their career. Always get plenty of recommendations and screen candidates carefully.

Family Daycare Homes

Almost 40 percent of infants and toddlers in a daycare setting are enrolled in family daycare homes. Family daycare is offered in the home of the primary provider, who usually has up to six children of varying ages in her care. Many new parents like the intimacy and affordability of family daycare.

Many family daycare homes are part of a network of childcare resource and referral agencies. Some are part of human service organizations. Childcare resource centers are listed in your phone book. They offer information about which daycare homes in their network have openings, where they are located, what they charge, and whether they are registered or licensed.

ADVANTAGES OF FAMILY DAYCARE HOMES

- Childcare occurs in a natural, home setting.
- Family daycare homes are often inexpensive.
- Mixed-age groups allow children interactions through a variety of socialization experiences.
- One consistent caregiver forms a relationship with your infant.
- Some providers offer flexible weekend and evening hours.
- Many are licensed or registered with the State.

DISADVANTAGES OF FAMILY DAYCARE HOMES

- Alternative care may be unavailable if the provider is sick or on vacation.
- They are harder to monitor for quality of care.
- Some are not licensed or registered.
- Children are exposed to illness.

When considering the options of a family daycare home, be just as clear in your expectations and priorities as you would be at a "commercial" facility. Exercise your right to ask the provider these questions:

- Is your home licensed or registered?
- What is your policy on the handling and storage of breastmilk?
- Is space available to breastfeed my baby?
- How many children are in your care?
- Do you have backup support during your own family illness or vacation?
- Do you transport children in an insured vehicle? Do you have a valid driver's license?
- Are car seats available?
- Are you trained in CPR and first aid?
- What are your policies on discipline, emergencies, inclement weather, dispensing medications, and sick children?
- Can my baby still attend if he is ill?
- Is there still a charge if my infant is absent from daycare?
- What are your hours of operation? Do you offer flexible hours?
- What is the cost?

Interview likely candidates more than once, and have your baby available for at least one of the interviews to observe his interaction with the provider and the provider's ease with your infant. Many babies need time to get used to someone else, but at least you'll get a preview of what you can expect.

Commercial Daycare

Most commercial or formal daycare centers are licensed facilities that meet State health and safety standards. Generally speaking, most daycares don't permit infants any younger than six weeks old. So if you need to return to work sooner than six weeks after birth, you may need an alternative.

Consider the following as you list your priorities and do your research.

ADVANTAGES OF DAYCARE CENTERS

- They are often licensed or registered with the State.
- Staff are often certified in CPR and first aid.
- Staff often hold early childhood degrees or receive specialized training in child development.
- Enrichment programs are offered for older babies.
- There are opportunities for babies to interact and socialize.
- Care is monitored by other staff and the daycare director.

DISADVANTAGES OF DAYCARE CENTERS

- Children are often exposed to illness from other babies.
- Noisy, busy environments can overstimulate babies.
- Having several providers can be confusing to your infant.
- Hours usually range from 6:00 A.M. to 6:00 P.M., without flexibility.
- Staff turnover is often high.
- Formal daycare centers are expensive.

In addition to the question listed above for family daycare, ask the formal daycare center providers these questions:

- Are activities structured or are they child-driven?
- How many children are cared for by each provider?
- How long have the current staff members been in place?
- Is there clear communication between the center providers and parents in the form of conferences, flyers, or parent groups?

As you tour the center, pay special attention to the atmosphere and activities. Are rooms and toys clean and inviting? Are children engaged in developmentally appropriate activities? Do children seem happy? Are crying babies attended to and soothed? Is the environment clean and safe for young children?

Ask for references from other parents with infants the same age as your baby. Call them and ask them to describe the quality of care their babies receive in the center, as well as the pros and cons of placing children in this center's care. When you enroll, ask for copies of all policies and procedures, and get a copy of your contract. Daycare is a business deal. Enter into it carefully.

Dollars and Sense

There's no doubt about it: Most childcare is pricey. Consider the following information about the costs of each option:

- **Family care:** This can be free or low cost. Just remember that you might get exactly what you pay for. Even if a family member begs to babysit for free, you might consider insisting on a pay rate to keep the arrangement professional.
- **Au pairs:** The weekly cost of an au pair is not as much as other childcare, but there are hidden costs. There is the agency fee and the fee for health insurance for the au pair, not to mention basic room and board, and additional expenses when you include your au pair on family vacations. Sometimes you must pay an au pair's round-trip airfare from their home country.
- **Nannies:** Nannies may cost the same or a bit less than daycare. However, the price may be the same for one child as for two or three. There is also less likelihood that the nanny will charge based on the age of the child.
- **Daycare:** Daycare costs will depend on whether it is a chain or a large daycare versus a family-run daycare (which is usually the cheaper option). You may also receive cost breaks as your baby gets older.

Tax Tips and Flex Accounts

There are certain tax incentives available relating to childcare expenses. What type and how much of an incentive it really is depends on many factors, including the cost of child care and your annual combined income.

Smart Mama Tricks: **Save on Childcare with an FSA**

With a Flexible Spending Account (FSA), you choose the amount you wish to set aside for dependent care by taking a pretax portion out of each paycheck. You then apply to receive these funds back over the course of the year.

Tax law changes frequently. Contact your tax advisor or the Internal Revenue Service (IRS) about the actual amount of deductions and what type of childcare qualifies.

Chapter 17

Fun with Food

For some reason, first-time moms often have an urge to start solids early. Well, there are those cute little feeding bibs, tiny white spoons, and Peter Rabbit bowls just staring at you from the shelf, and it's hard to wait to play with these new toys. What fun to see your baby light up in surprise at a new taste and lean forward to slurp up every drop! (Or not—like when your baby knocks the spoon onto the floor and then spits all over you.)

What's the Rush?

As your baby grows, she'll eventually become ready for solid food. Exactly when this happens varies greatly from one child to another. In many societies around the world, infants are not introduced to solid food until after nine to twelve months. Yet just a generation ago, our American mothers were encouraged to begin adding rice cereal to the baby bottle at as early as six weeks (a practice that is now strongly discouraged).

There seems to be as much variation among experts and physicians on when to start solids. Today, some doctors are okay with exclusive breastfeeding for as long as one year if your baby continues to thrive on breastmilk alone and shows no interest in solid food. However, most doctors say that babies are ready to eat some solid food at four to six months when their digestive tract is fully developed and when they are beginning to sit without support. The AAP recommends breastfeeding exclusively until the age of six months and that your baby continue to breastfeed for at least one year.

 Smart Mama Tricks: **Preserve the "Virgin Gut"**

Once your breastfed infant ingests formula or solid food, the microbial makeup of her gut changes. Exclusively breastfed babies have increased numbers of good bacteria and decreased numbers of bad bacteria when compared with babies who are fed formula even intermittently. These "virgin guts" are thought to reduce the risk of illness and allergies in your baby's early months of life.

Other Reasons for Waiting

By about six months most babies are physically ready to swallow solid foods. The so-called tongue extrusion reflex, in which most things that go into a baby's mouth are quickly pushed out by her tongue, fades away. An older baby's digestive enzymes have matured to the point where she can fairly efficiently break down solid foods.

Her digestive tract has completed a maturation process known as "closure," preventing potentially allergenic substances from entering the bloodstream. It's important to wait for these capacities to develop, because once a breastfed baby starts solids, she may lose some of her protection against infections and allergies.

- She's at least six months old (if breastfed) or at least four months old (if bottle-fed)
- She imitates a vulture when you're eating, ready to pounce on your food
- She stops sticking her tongue out when her mouth is touched
- She sits with support and controls her head well enough to lean forward when she wants more food
- She's starting to sit up on her own
- She can communicate that she's full
- She drinks more than 32 to 40 ounces of formula, or breastfeeds more frequently, possibly more than ten times a day, and still wants more
- She's at least twice her birth weight or at least 13 to 15 pounds

 Smart Mama Tricks: **Learn Your Baby's Appetites**

Some babies do better eating solids before they eat anything else, when they are the most hungry. Others get frustrated taking small amounts of food off of a spoon when they are so hungry, and they do better eating solids after breastmilk or formula or at a separate time altogether. Learn the best time for your child's solid food feedings.

What's on the Menu?

Iron-fortified rice cereal is the most recommended first meal because it is easily absorbed by the body and is one of the least allergenic foods. There are many brands of precooked powdered dry cereal, including a few made from organic brown rice. Mix these cereals with breastmilk or formula until the consistency is watery, but still sticks to the spoon. The familiar taste of the breastmilk or formula will help your baby adjust to eating solids.

FIRST FEEDING TIPS

- Feed your baby when she is hungry, but not extremely hungry. If she is too hungry, she might become confused and upset by your offer of something unfamiliar when all she wants is the breast or her bottle.
- Feed your baby early in the day (midmorning is best), so that you can watch for any adverse reactions as the day goes on.
- Don't feed your baby more than a few tablespoons in the first few feedings, even if she is excited and eating well. Overindulgence may very well lead to an uncomfortable overfull tummy and indigestion.
- Watch your baby for signs that she is finished eating. She might turn her head away or wave away the spoon. Let her set the pace.
- Remember the "rule of fist." Your baby's stomach is about the size of her tiny fist. If she eats a tablespoon of cereal followed by a full feeding of breastmilk, she will be satisfied.

It's All in the Wrist

For your baby's first supper, pick a time when she's starting to seem hungry, but not frantically so. Make sure she is basically upright, with her head tipped slightly back.

Scoop a tiny bit of cereal on an infant or demitasse spoon—or even your own clean finger—and put it just into the front of your baby's mouth. Don't shove it in; she needs to learn for herself how to get the food off of the spoon and far enough back into her mouth to swallow. Since you're introducing this at a stage when she is mouthing everything in sight, she'll probably open her mouth as soon as the spoon gets close.

Smart Mama Tricks: **The Puppet Trick**

Use a hand puppet to grasp the spoon for feeding your baby. This is so funny to some babies that it actually distracts from eating, but others are fascinated and happily accept food from their new friend. (A bath-toy hand puppet works best because it's easy to clean.)

Then let your baby do whatever she wants with the cereal. She may try to suck the spoon. She may push the cereal out with her tongue. At this point, you may decide that she's not ready and try again another time. Or, you can matter-of-factly scoop it off of her chin and back into her mouth. Eventually, she may swallow and then open her mouth for another bite. Once she turns away, she's had enough, even if it's only been a few spoonfuls. Respect her appetite and stop when she's full; don't try to coax in one last bite. Let your baby decide how much she wants to eat. Learning to eat only when she feels hungry and to stop when she feels full are healthy habits that should continue into adulthood.

Fun with Food

Life after Rice Cereal

Introduce foods slowly and one at a time. Allow at least three days between introductions so you can identify potential problems. If you have a family history of food allergies, pay special attention to your baby's reactions to new foods.

Smart Mama Tricks: When Not to Make Your Own

Certain vegetables, such as beets, carrots, green beans, squash, turnips, spinach, or collard greens may contain nitrates from the soil in which they were grown. These nitrates can cause anemia in your baby. Don't prepare your own baby food from these particular vegetables. Commercial baby food manufacturers are required to test for these nitrates, so you may safely buy these vegetables already prepared.

Pureed Vegetables

Join the "vegetables first" crowd. Babies already have a preference for sweets, so fruits will be readily accepted. Some vegetables, on the other hand, might take getting used to. Your baby might refuse to eat vegetables if fruits are introduced first. Baby vegetables come pureed or strained.

One to two tablespoons per day is all your baby needs for the next three months. Add one new vegetable per week.

Pureed Fruits

Fruits are almost always enthusiastically explored and accepted by babies. Fruits without added sugars are best, so mash peaches canned in their own juice or grate a fresh pear. As with vegetables, one to two tablespoons of fruit per day is all a baby needs for healthy development. Add one new fruit per week.

Meats

Meats are important sources of iron and protein, making pureed meats a good choice for early foods. You can buy jarred meats, or you can simply save a few tablespoons of the unseasoned fully cooked ground meat you're fixing for dinner and mash it well for your baby.

Eggs should be cooked and all egg whites removed. Egg whites are a known allergen. Hard boil an egg and serve the cooled, mashed yolk.

 Smart Mama Tricks: **Use Two Spoons**

Use a separate spoon for taking food out of the baby food jar. If you use the same spoon that goes into baby's mouth, saliva and bacteria from the spoon will contaminate the leftover food in the jar.

Dairy

Wait until your baby is at least twelve months old before feeding her dairy products. The protein in cow's milk can be difficult to break down and can cause allergies in young babies. Cow's milk is also a poor source of iron, unlike breastmilk and formula.

Juice

You can introduce juice at around six to eight months of age, but many doctors prefer that you feed pureed or mashed fruit, which is loaded with valuable fiber, instead of juice.

The AAP's Committee on Nutrition reports that when you offer juice before solid foods are introduced, you risk juice replacing breastmilk or formula in your baby's diet, which can result in lowering baby's intake of protein, fats, vitamins, and minerals like iron, calcium, and zinc.

Smart Mama Tricks: Limit Juice

In the case of juice, more is not always better. Because it can cause rapid tooth decay due to its high natural sugar content, feed juice only in a cup, not from a bottle, and establish a regular toothbrushing routine. Juice may be linked to obesity, so limit its use to no more than four to six ounces a day. Avoid "juice drinks," which may contain little actual juice and loads of added sugar.

I Need a Drink!

You can begin teaching your baby to drink from a cup at about the same time you start solids, or even a little sooner. Offer sips of breastmilk or formula from a cup beginning at about five months—not for nutrition, but for practice. Put the cup to her lips and tip it until just a tiny sip pours out.

There are three basic kind of infant cups, and you'll eventually want to get your baby used to all three of them. She should learn to drink from a cup without a top, controlling the flow with her lips. You will also want her to drink occasionally from a cup with a spouted lid: for example, when she's eating finger foods in her highchair and you want her to have a drink available, but don't want her to soak herself if you step away. Then there are times for a no-spill cup. These cups have valves inside their spouts, and don't spill even if shaken. They're great for the stroller and the car.

Let There Be Lumps!

At eight to ten months or more, many babies will be pretty proficient at slurping and swallowing, and you'll be used to the routine.

Then your baby pulls a fast one. "No more mush!" her pursed lips seem to say as she knocks the spoon out of your hand and pureed carrots spatter across the floor. Your baby is sick of goop.

However, she has only a few teeth—and is not nearly ready to handle a knife and fork. You can't expect to pass her the steak and potatoes just yet. (Well, maybe the potatoes.)

One Lump or Two?

One option is moving to lumpier baby foods. The prepared versions are marked Stage Three or designated for older babies. If you are making them yourself, don't puree them as long and leave in some chunks. The change in texture and the more complex tastes of these foods may get your little bird opening her mouth again.

Or not. Some kids are used to slurping baby mush, and food for older babies makes them gag and frequently throw up much of their meal. They may be ready for something to get their teeth or gums into, and the mushy/chewy combination can be too confusing for them. What's a parent to do?

 Smart Mama Tricks: **Learn the Art of Camouflage**

Dip your baby's spoon into the less-favored food first, then dip it into a food she finds more appealing. Many pounds of mashed peas have been consumed in this way, cloaked in pureed peaches.

Cereal Strategies

Grab the Cheerios, or, to be brand neutral, oat cereal rings. Scatter a few on your baby's tray, and she'll try to pick them up and put them in her mouth. These may entertain her enough for you to slip in a few spoonfuls of mush in between bites.

Another option is a teething biscuit. There are a number of varieties available, or you can make your own. Read the labels; some have a lot more sugar than others. Teething biscuits dissolve into mush as your baby gums them. (But don't leave your baby alone with one—or alone eating anything at this stage—since large pieces can break off and pose a choking danger.)

Smart Mama Tricks: **If at First You Don't Succeed ...**

Sometimes babies take a while to warm up to a new food—sometimes a long, long while. Continue to offer it up to fifteen different times; and maybe on that fifteenth time, your baby will surprise you by finally taking a bite. Meanwhile, space your attempts several days or a week apart, and don't make a fuss if the food is refused.

Allergy Alert

Approximately 3 to 7 percent of adults and children experience allergies to food. You may already know that your baby is prone to food allergies. Perhaps food allergies run in one or both parents' families, or your baby may have even displayed allergic reactions to foods transmitted to her in her mother's milk. However, this is often not the case, and an allergic reaction may take parents by surprise.

If you suspect a food allergy, discuss it with your child's pediatrician. The doctor will probably recommend you keep close track of what your child is eating and its relationship to the onset of symptoms. Keep in mind that all of these symptoms can also indicate an illness, like a virus or infection. Even if your baby developed a symptom right after you started a new food, it could still be just a coincidence, so talk to your pediatrician if you think your baby is developing a food allergy or intolerance. This is especially important before you make big changes to her diet or begin restricting a lot of different foods.

SIGNS OF FOOD ALLERGIES

- Runny nose, watery eyes, sneezing
- Diaper rash or rash around the anus
- Rash, especially on the face
- Swollen lips, hands, or feet
- Hives
- Sores in the mouth
- Headache
- Asthma, bronchitis, or recurrent ear infections
- Nausea, diarrhea, vomiting, or gas
- Poor weight gain
- Fatigue
- Unusual or irritable behavior

Certain foods are more likely to trigger allergic reactions in some babies. You may want to introduce these later, rather than sooner. If you or someone in your immediate family has a particular food allergy, discuss this with your provider before you introduce this food into your baby's diet. Be alert for reactions if you try any of these following foods and consider waiting until baby is a year old before introducing them:

- Citrus fruits, tomatoes, strawberries
- Wheat, corn, soy products
- Egg whites, cow's milk

- Shellfish
- Peanuts

Food Hazards

The following foods can be dangerous to young kids, whose bodies and swallowing techniques are not fully formed:

- Babies who are younger than one year should not eat honey, because it contains bacterial spores that may cause clostridium botulism, a potentially fatal illness.
- Any hard or chunky piece of food is a potential choking hazard. Among other things, avoid: popcorn, whole berries, candy, raw carrots and apples, seeds in fruit or olives, nuts, grapes (unless cut into very small pieces), or any hard-baked goods like pretzels.
- Peanut butter and other nut butters can cause choking if taken in large bites.

 Smart Mama Tricks: **Try Frozen Veggies**

Keep a few bags of frozen vegetables in your freezer. You can prepare small amounts for baby, as needed, without worrying about spoilage as you would with fresh. Contrary to popular belief, frozen vegetables often have more nutrients than fresh, because the nutrient value has not been degraded through distribution and handling.

Healthy Habits

Early infancy is probably the time when you have the most control over what your child eats. After all, a nine-month-old can't go to the pantry to get a cookie or to the refrigerator to get a soda. Sure, she might cry if she doesn't get what she wants, but you still have control over what you give her to eat. And at this point, she won't miss what she hasn't yet tasted.

♡ Take Care of You: One Meal for Everyone

Once the food introduction period is over, try to get your baby to eat the same meals as the rest of your family. You don't want to get stuck in the rut of preparing two different dishes at every meal. Once baby eats what you eat, whether you're cutting it into small chunks or you're still beating it to a pulp, you'll spend less time in the kitchen.

One of the biggest sources of junk food in an infant's diet is the type of finger foods you give her to snack on. Avoid sugary cereals and other typical junk foods, such as cookies, chips, or doughnuts. Better options include soft, small pieces of fruits and vegetables, whole-grain toast or pasta, and low-sugar cereals.

Chapter 18

Movin' and Groovin'

Your baby is only three days old, but clearly she's a genius. She already knows how to grab your finger and move her feet like she's walking. Well, okay, those are just reflexes. But hey, wasn't that a smile? Although babies don't smile in response to your smile until two months or so, you may catch a few smiles from a newborn.

All Babies Are Different

Many babies reach certain milestones around the same age, while some jump ahead or fall behind the "norm." If this is your first child, you'll be eager to fill in that list, noting when she first rolls over, sits up, and crawls. If this is your second or third baby, you'll probably have mixed feelings when she hits a milestone. You'll be applauding her achievement, but will be aware of how much it will change your life. (A baby who turns over is no longer easy to diaper; a baby who crawls needs a childproofed house.) And you may be mourning the passing of an earlier stage.

First mom or experienced mom, you'll be noting your baby's developmental milestones, and, whether you plan to or not, comparing them to those of your baby's peers. Odds are she'll do some things earlier than others, some things later, and once in a while will hit the median. You may be running to Home Depot for safety gates months earlier than you had expected or wondering why your baby hasn't taken a step while other babies her age are jogging. She may be focused on learning to talk and will get to walking later. However she's progressing, don't forget that there is a wide range of "normal." All babies are different. Crawling, walking, or talking earlier does not necessarily indicate greater intelligence, athleticism, or health.

♡ Take Care of You: Live in the Moment

Instead of always looking ahead to what's next, enjoy today's stage of development (and take photos); it may not last until tomorrow.

Milestones

No milestone chart can tell you what your baby will—or should—be doing at a particular age. Indeed, child development experts differ in their opinions of when milestones can occur. And then those opinions change. View this chart as a general, loose guideline.

Now that babies are put to sleep on their backs, you'll need to place baby on her stomach for short periods of time when she is awake. (If your baby cries the whole time that she is on her tummy, limit each time to just a few minutes or wait several days and then try again.)

Again, try not to compare babies of the same age. Do talk to your pediatrician if you are truly concerned that your baby isn't meeting her milestones.

Motor Milestones

AGE	MILESTONE
Birth–1 month	side-to-side head turn
2–4 months	mini-pushup
2–5 months	swipes at object
2–5 months	brings both hands together
3–7 months	rolls over
3–7 months	grasps objects
5–9 months	sits unsupported
6–12 months	crawls (or somehow travels on four limbs)
7–13 months	pulls up to a stand
8–17 months	walks

Language Milestones

AGE	MILESTONE
newborn	cries
1–2 months	cries differently to communicate pain, hunger, and exhaustion
6 weeks–2 months	coos or oohs (vowels)
4–5 months	understands his name
4–8 months	babbles (consonants)
9 months	understands "no"
10–12 months	babbles without repeating syllables
8–14 months	points
10 months	responds to a spoken request
10–18 months	says first words

Your One-Toothed Wonder

The average infant gets her first tooth at about six months, but the timing of this event varies quite a bit. You can generally expect that your baby will get her first tooth sometime between three and fifteen months.

Is She Teething or Is She Sick?

Most parents suspect that their baby is teething at around three or four months when she starts drooling a lot and wants to chew on things. While it is possible for a baby to get her first tooth that early, in most cases those aren't signs of teething. Instead, those are normal milestones that most children begin at this age, whether or not they are teething.

Still, your baby may start drooling more and want to chew on things when she really does start teething. Look for other teething signs and symptoms. Can you see or feel her first tooth coming through? Do her gums look red or swollen? Mild irritability, crying, a low-grade temperature (not over 100 degrees Fahrenheit), excessive drooling, and chewing on fingers or anything hard are occasional signs of teething. If your baby has a higher fever, runny nose, cough, or diarrhea, don't be quick to attribute it to teething. Treat those symptoms as possibly relating to a different condition and see your provider, if appropriate.

After your baby gets her first tooth, she'll usually continue to get three or four more teeth every three or four months. This will continue until she gets all twenty of her baby teeth at around two and a half years old.

Brushing Baby Teeth

You don't necessarily need to brush these first teeth, but you do need to clean them. A moist washcloth or a piece of soft gauze can be used to wipe them clean before bed each night. Once your child gets several more teeth, you can begin using a soft infant's toothbrush instead.

Smart Mama Tricks: Make Toothbrushing Fun

Babies love to imitate. Brush your teeth in front of your baby before you try to brush his teeth. Name your baby's teeth and sing to them while you brush. Look for something silly hiding behind her teeth.

You probably don't need to start using toothpaste until your baby gets a few more teeth. And once you do, be sure to use a non-fluoride toothpaste until your child is old enough to spit out the paste. Swallowing too much of a fluoride toothpaste can cause fluorosis and staining on her teeth.

Damage Control

In addition to coughs, sniffles, and sneezes, you'll have to deal with the bumps and bruises your baby will inevitably encounter despite your best efforts. She'll be increasingly exposed once she's mobile, but even infants can get bumped, burned, or scratched.

First Things First

Before you buy a lot of childproofing gear, do the simple things. Gather up any poisonous items, from detergent to vitamins, and put them on your highest shelves (locking a cabinet works only if you always remember to close the lock). Cut looped blind cords into separate strands to reduce the choking hazard, or knot them up out of reach. Make sure you can identify all your houseplants (if you have to, take a leaf to a local garden center) and confirm that they are nontoxic. Turn your water heater down to 120 degrees Fahrenheit, if you haven't already. Put at least one trash can in a locked cabinet, and think before you throw things into accessible trash cans (avoid things like empty containers of cleaning products or used disposable razors).

Make a list of the childproofing gear you need to get. Don't buy everything in sight; you may be wasting your money, since some babies have no interest in toilets, doorstoppers, or stereo cords.

BASIC CHILDPROOFING FOR CRAWLERS

- Cover electrical outlets.
- Remove or block access to easily tipped over furniture (like lamps).
- Move breakables or other dangerous knickknacks out of reach.
- Regularly hunt for dropped coins or other potential choking hazards.
- Hide, coil, cover, or block access to electrical cords.
- Knot blind cords out of reach, or cut through loop.
- Install gates both at the top and bottom of each staircase.
- Do not use a baby walker anywhere around stairs (better yet, do not use a baby walker, period).

- Cede the lower shelves of your bookcases to your child; move your books out of reach, and restock shelves with baby books.
- Place a heat-resistant safety gate around the fireplace.
- Make sure your pool, if you have one, is solidly fenced and the gate is kept closed and locked. Hot tubs should be kept closed and locked when not in use, and toilets should be locked. Don't even leave a pail of water unattended.

 Smart Mama Tricks: **Poison-Control Hotline**

Post this toll-free Poison Control hotline number by every telephone in the house: 1-800-222-1222. In an emergency, a poison-safety expert will help you figure out what to do for your child.

ADDITIONAL CHILDPROOFING FOR CRUISERS AND WALKERS
- Install window guards if you live in an apartment or house with multiple floors.
- Lock kitchen cabinets and drawers that contain anything dangerous (knives, etc.).
- Turn pot handles toward the back of the stove when cooking and install stove knob guards.
- Make sure bookcases and other furniture will not topple over.
- Secure the TV so it won't fall if tugged on or pushed.
- Place nonskid backing on rugs that your child might slip or slide on.

Movin' and Groovin'

- Set the temperature of hot water heaters to 120 degrees Fahrenheit.
- Install childproof doorknob covers on doors leading to the outside, particularly the door leading to the garage (often one of the most dangerous rooms in the house).

Always keep an eye on your mobile baby; you never know what they can get into!

Choking Prevention

Parents often worry about their baby choking on food once she starts finger and table foods, but the average house has a lot of other choke hazards that put babies even more at risk. These hazards can range from large pieces of food to coins your infant may find on the floor to your older children's toys.

Smart Mama Tricks: Choking First Aid

First aid for a choking infant usually involves placing the baby face down on your lap and giving five back blows with the heel of your hand to the area just between the infant's shoulder blades. If that doesn't work, the next step is placing the infant face up and giving five compressions to the infant's breastbone. Take a CPR class to learn how to do this correctly.

Younger children naturally put everything in their mouths. This is the way that they learn to explore the world around them, so it is impossible to "teach" them not to put things in their mouths. Instead, it is the parents' responsibility to keep the house free of choking hazards—which can be a daily chore.

Make sure you call 911 for help, even if you do dislodge whatever was in your baby's throat. You can't know what damage may have already been done.

Raining Cats and Dogs

Your dog may have simply issued some cursory sniffs when you brought your infant home, and pricked up his ears (or ran and hid) when baby's trademark wail ensued. But once your child is mobile, to your pet she becomes an entirely different animal.

Proper Pet Etiquette

The basic rule of thumb: Never leave your baby and pet together unattended. It's a good rule to follow. Baby could crawl over to kitty, grab a handful of fur, and end up with a sharp-clawed swat in the face.

In the meantime, start teaching your child proper pet etiquette as soon as she takes notice of your animals. Even if you have the sweetest, most tolerant dog or cat on the planet, when you consider that there are an estimated 65 million pet dogs and 77 million pet cats in the United States, your baby will undoubtedly encounter many other pets throughout her childhood. The better prepared she is, the less likely she'll ever get hurt.

Gentle Touches

Once your baby can get her hands on your pet, she'll likely pat (at best) and grab and yank (at worst). Teach your child "gentle touches," repeating the words while you demonstrate the correct way to smoothly stroke your pet from front to back, in the direction that the fur grows. ("Gentle touches" works well when your baby starts to play with other children, too.) Avoid petting the head and tail for now—animal eyes and ears and noses are too tempting for toddlers, as is a tail to pull.

Give your dog a quiet place it can retreat to that is away from probing little hands. Teach your toddler that when doggie goes to his bed or crate or corner, it must be left alone—especially when sleeping. Cats tend to find their own hideouts where they can't be reached, under furniture or up on high shelves. Still, teach your children not to follow, chase, or tease the kitty.

Mealtime Danger

For dogs, mealtime is often a highly charged situation. Don't combine an inquisitive, crawling baby with a hungry dog at its dish unless you're looking for trouble. Keep baby and dog separated at feeding time.

Chapter 19

Your Brave New World

Once your baby arrived, you were probably longing for your life to go back to normal. But the truth is, your life never goes back to the way it was before giving birth. You have to instead find your new normal. If you're like most new moms, your first year of motherhood is the most exhausting, all-encompassing, heartbreaking, and rewarding year of your life. There are the sleepless nights that wear you out, crying jags (yours and the baby's) that threaten to send you over the edge, scary head bumps that rush you to the pediatrician, and gooey diaper blowouts of unimaginable proportions. Meanwhile, you've been constantly adjusting and fine-tuning your parenting skills. And maybe you're even thinking about having another baby.

Desperate Housewife?

Yes, there is a life after baby. You can successfully be a mother and a wife, though some fine-tuning may be necessary. Priorities shift, free time shrinks, spontaneity issues arise, and generally, life is different now. It will take some effort on both your and your mate's part to make your relationship work with a new baby in the house.

Date Nights

Date nights are simply times you carve out of your hectic life to be alone with your partner. This is a foreign concept to most postpartum families. But it will help you continue to strengthen your relationship with your partner.

♡ Take Care of You: Your Body Is a Temple

Don't forget to treat your body well. Consider a manicure, pedicure, or massage to give yourself a boost and help you feel attractive. Often these simple things can really boost your body image. You haven't lost it forever; it's just hidden.

Dates don't have to happen at night or even on the weekend. A date for you and your partner can simply consist of a few uninterrupted hours together. You can sit and talk over a quiet dinner out or curl up on your couch to watch television. Don't fold laundry or even answer the phone.

You may choose a time when your baby is sleeping to reconnect with your partner. This way, you don't have to hire help for the baby, but if the baby wakes up, this will certainly distract you from your date. Do whatever you can to limit distractions during these intimate times.

Alone Time

You may find it hard to believe that your baby is not permanently connected to your hip. It's perfectly acceptable to get out of your house without taking anyone with you. "Alone" takes on a whole new meaning once you're a mom. There will be days when you may consider begging your partner to watch the baby while you go to the grocery store alone. Once you start viewing the grocery store as a hot hangout, it's time to get out alone more often.

The Parent You Want to Be

You probably have an idea of how you want to mother your child over the years to come—perhaps drawing on a combination of your own life experiences and role models. Or maybe you remember what you judged to be poor decisions on the part of your own parents and hope to escape committing them yourself. No matter what kind of parenting guidelines you have set for yourself, remember that things will always change as your baby grows.

Your Childhood

When you were growing up, did you keep a running list of all the things your parents did that you would never, ever do to your children? As you grew older, you probably realized that your parents didn't do as bad a job as you once thought. After all, they raised you, didn't they?

While it's certainly a good idea to learn from your own less-than-perfect childhood experiences, remember that your vision at the time may have been skewed. Kids often overreact when they are young, and no one likes being told what to do. You'll soon realize that there are many ways of teaching a child to be safe and confident in this world.

Just keep in mind that just like your folks, you too will make mistakes as a parent. Pointing out and explaining your mistakes to your child enables him to accept his own mistakes and learn from them, too. Just as you did, your child will realize one day that even parents are only human.

Parenting with a Partner

Sometimes the hardest part of parenting isn't deciding how you want to parent; it's hashing out a parenting philosophy that works for both you and your partner. When the two of you agree, chances are things will go smoothly—you won't have to argue and debate every time it comes to making a decision about your baby's needs. Having the same thoughts helps present a united front in parenting, something that's important as your child grows up.

This is a partnership. Talk to each other and figure out if you have similar goals. Maybe you have the same goals, just different approaches. If you both believe that your child should learn to respect his elders, how do you intend to achieve this? One of you might believe that constant reinforcement by encouraging your child to say respectful things is best, while the other may believe that role modeling respect is the key. Eke out time to read parenting and child-development books together—or attend parenting classes if they are offered in your area.

Another Baby?

You've probably been getting too much sleep if you're already thinking about another baby! Or maybe the sight of your once tiny newborn blowing out his first birthday candle has you craving an infant again. But then, as you watch your sleeping toddler's eyelids flutter and his tummy rise and fall with breath, you sigh and wonder if it's humanly possible to love anything in this world as much as you love your firstborn.

Love Enough for Two

In truth, your love expands with the number of children you have. Don't worry about loving your babies equally, but love them differently as the unique individuals they are. The second child may not get that intense two-parent, 100 percent focus your first child did, especially if you space your babies close together. But the new baby will have the added bonus of a sibling to entertain and interact with him, which enriches his life experience in a different way.

Age Differences

There are as many opinions on the ideal spacing between children as there are people to ask. There are benefits and disadvantages to having kids close in age or far apart. Obviously, if you have them close together, you can get the high-needs parenting and diaper duty over all at once, but you may be paying double for daycare or preschool costs (not to mention college).

The closer together your children are, the fewer baby items you can reuse, because the first child is still using them. You may have to buy an additional big-ticket item or two, such as a car seat and a crib.

Too much time between babies means you will have to get used to all the "baby stuff" again, such as sleepless nights, diapers, and breast- or bottle-feeding. An older first child might resent losing out on his "only child" status more if she has longer to get used to being an "only," or conversely she might be happy to entertain and help care for younger sibs. Keep in mind that children spaced far apart will have different needs, such as an older child needing rides to school and soccer practice while the younger child needs his regular naps.

Then there's yourself to think about. Do you want to go through a pregnancy and caring for a newborn while you're still chasing a toddler around? Or are you feeling your age and thinking that it's now or never? If you had a cesarean birth, your provider may have advised you to wait at least eighteen months before becoming pregnant again. Furthermore, a recent study published in the *Journal of the American Medical Association* (*JAMA*) concluded that inter-pregnancy intervals (the time span between the delivery of one baby and the conception of the next) shorter than eighteen months and longer than fifty-nine months are associated with increased risk of low birth weight, small size for gestational age, and pre-term birth.

The decision to have another baby, just as the choice to have the first one, is highly personal and individual. Play scientist. Observe your friends who have more than one child. Ask everyone their opinions. Most important, talk to your partner and determine what you both want for your family.

You Did It!

You gain so much confidence as you experience new things with your baby. Many times you don't even realize what you've gained over the course of a year. You've learned not only to give birth to a new human being, but to care for her and raise her from a tiny, helpless creature to an independence-striving toddler.

> ## ♡ Take Care of You: **Adjust Your Expectations**
>
> *As a mother, sometimes you will consider your day a success if everyone is alive at the end of it. Don't let this shake your confidence; it's all a matter of perspective. It's a good day when you say it is.*

In the early days and weeks, you may have been unsure of your decisions as a parent. Perhaps for the first time, you realized that you and your partner alone were completely responsible for another human being. You made careful choices according to your and your family's needs, and you learned from your mistakes. You have become the perfect mother for your baby, warts and all.

Sometime during this first year, you may have learned to gulp your food, shoveling it into your mouth as fast as you could before baby started to fuss, putting an end to dinner. When you can, remember to slow down. Chew. Put your fork down between bites. Taste the meal. And this goes for everything in your baby's early years—slow down, pay attention, and enjoy what you and your child are doing. Love your new life. Don't rush. It will be over all too soon.

In the years to come, whether they're wearing their cap and gown, getting married, or having babies of their own, you'll never forget what they looked like, what they felt like—what you felt like—when you held them in your arms this magical first year.

Appendix

Resources

Pregnancy Resources

The following are Web sites, books, and organizations that can help you through the trials and tribulations of pregnancy.

PREGNANCY WEB SITES

About Pregnancy Guide
http://pregnancy.about.com
This Web site offers pregnancy-related articles, a pregnancy calendar, ultrasound photos, community support, a belly gallery, and other pregnancy-related items and information.

Childbirth.org
www.childbirth.org
This pregnancy Web site is dedicated to helping you maintain a healthy pregnancy. There are many informative articles on all aspects of pregnancy, and fun programs, including a boy-or-girl quiz and a birth-plan creator.

Lamaze Institute for Normal Birth
normalbirth.lamaze.org
Here you'll find great information on having a healthy, normal birth. This includes the researched, linked six care practices that are considered to be the cornerstone of a healthy birth.

BOOKS ON PREGNANCY

The Pregnancy Book by William Sears, M.D., and Martha Sears, R.N., I.B.C.L.C.
This doctor/nurse, husband/wife team gives the facts about pregnancy and birth. The book is laid out in a convenient month-by-month format to help you find the information you need, when you need it.

The Thinking* Woman's *Guide to a Better Birth by Henci Goer
Ms. Goer gives you all the medical information in layman's terms to help you decide the safest, healthiest way for your baby to be born.

American Academy of Husband Coached Childbirth (Bradley Method)
P.O. Box 5224
Sherman Oaks, CA 91413-5224
800-4-A-BIRTH
www.bradleybirth.com
The Bradley Method of childbirth includes the use of deep relaxation and breathing with the help of the husband or partner through the labor process. The classes emphasize prenatal nutrition and exercise and their influence on a healthy pregnancy.

American Academy of Pediatrics (AAP)
141 Northwest Point Boulevard
Elk Grove Village, IL 60007
847-434-4000
www.aap.org
The AAP is the leading authority on children's issues and the governing body of pediatricians across America.

American College of Nurse Midwives (ACNM)
818 Connecticut Avenue, NW, Suite 900
Washington, DC 20006
Phone: 202-728-9860
Fax: 202-728-9897
www.midwife.org
ACNM certifies nurse midwives (CNM) throughout the United States. It focuses on the care of low-risk women through pregnancy and birth as well as other time periods of life. Well-woman care is their specialty.

American College of Obstetricians and Gynecologists (ACOG)
409 12th Street, SW
P.O. Box 96920
Washington, DC 20090-6920
www.acog.org
ACOG is the premiere organization for obstetricians and gynecologists. It manages the post-medical-school training and certification of this specialty. These physicians are trained in the care of the woman during all stages of life.

Coalition for Improving Maternity Services (CIMS)
P.O. Box 2346
Ponte Vedra Beach, FL 32004
888-282-CIMS
www.motherfriendly.org
CIMS has lots of great information on choosing a health-care provider and place of birth, as well as information on making decisions for yourself in pregnancy and beyond.

DONA International (Formerly Doulas of North America)
P.O. Box 626
Jasper, IN 47547
888-788-DONA
www.dona.org

DONA is the leading organization that certifies birth and postpartum doulas. A doula can assist the family before, during, or after birth. Using a doula has been shown to decrease the incidence of many complications in labor and postpartum, including cesarean section and postpartum depression.

International Cesarean Awareness Network (ICAN)
1304 Kingsdale Avenue
Redondo Beach, CA 90278
310-542-6400
www.ican-online.org
ICAN works toward the prevention of unnecessary cesareans and the emotional and physical recovery from cesareans.

International Childbirth Education Association (ICEA)
P.O. Box 20048
Minneapolis, MN 55420
952-854-8660
www.icea.org
]ICEA trains childbirth educators as well as prenatal fitness instructors throughout the world. Their Web site offers a search to help you find local instructors.

Lamaze International
2025 M Street, Suite 800
Washington, DC 20036-3309
202-367-1128
www.lamaze.org

Lamaze International is the leading certifying organization for childbirth educators. Promoting normal birth is the core of their philosophy as they train educators worldwide. Their site offers a directory, articles, and other interactive features.

Maternity Center Association
281 Park Avenue South, 5th Floor
New York, NY 10010
212-777-5000
www.maternitywise.org
Lots of great consumer advice can be found here. You can download new booklets on choosing cesarean birth, what you should know about vaginal birth after cesarean (VBAC), and more. There is even a complete pregnancy medical text available to read on their Web site.

Breastfeeding Resources
The following are helpful Web sites, books, and organizations with information and tips on breastfeeding.

WEB SITES
Breastfeeding Online
www.breastfeedingonline.com
This site has great information on breastfeeding, from how to start to how to deal with complications or issues that

Appendix

arise. You can also submit your questions and receive answers.

Growth Charts for the first year from the CDC
www.cdc.gov/growthcharts
These charts will help you track your baby's growth during the first year of his or her life.

The Nursing Mother's Companion by Kathleen Huggins
This breastfeeding book has a wealth of information that is broken down for ease of use. It also has a section on breastfeeding as a working mother, including pumps and pumping.

The Ultimate Breastfeeding Book of Answers by Dr. Jack Newman and Teresa Pitman
Pediatrician Dr. Newman and Teresa Pitman explain the benefits of breastfeeding, how to prevent problems with breastfeeding, and how to handle life as a breastfeeding mother.

International Lactation Consultant Association (ILCA)
1500 Sunday Drive, Suite 102
Raleigh, NC 27607
919-861-5577

www.ilca.org
ILCA certifies lactation consultants. Their Web site has information on finding a board-certified lactation consultant in your area, as well as information on how to become a board-certified lactation consultant.

La Leche League International
1400 N. Meacham Road
Schaumburg, IL 60173-4808
847-519-7730
www.lalecheleague.org
La Leche League provides information, education, and support for pregnant and breastfeeding women. There are monthly meetings held locally in many cities around the world, as well as a wealth of information via various publications. La Leche League also has some phone support available.

Pregnancy and Postpartum Fitness

Eat Well, Lose Weight while Breastfeeding by Eileen Behan
While breastfeeding does promote weight loss, the balance between keeping your baby well fed and losing weight can be a difficult one to maintain. Here's a different approach to the age-old

question of how you lose weight after pregnancy.

Essential Exercises for the Childbearing Year by Elizabeth Noble

Ms. Noble is a physical therapist, and the movement of the body is her specialty. She focuses on pregnancy fitness and howto stay healthy and fit while living a normal life during pregnancy. The book also includes information on proper body alignment and dealing with everyday questions like how to pick up older children.

The Everything® Pregnancy Fitness Book by Robin Elise Weiss

This book is a great overview of exercises for each trimester and the postpartum period. The photos are clear and the text succinct.

WEB SITES

Fit Pregnancy
www.fitpregnancy.com

Fit Pregnancy is based on a magazine of the same name. Here you will find pregnancy fitness- and wellness-related articles.

Walking Guide at About
http://walking.about.com

Your walking guide for every avenue of life. Includes the free ten-week Walk of Life program.

Managing Multiple Children Resources

BOOKS

Mothering Multiples by Karen Kerkoff Gromada, IBCLC

Not only is this advice indispensable, but it comes from the mother of twins! In this book you'll find lots of information on living with new twins (or more), from bringing them into the world to managing daily life. Also included are great sections on successfully feeding multiples, including premature babies.

WEB SITES

About Parenting of Multiples
http://multiples.about.com

This site starts at pregnancy and takes you through all the stages of physical, mental, and emotional development of multiples. There is also a gallery of photos of multiples, polls, and great articles on different aspects of raising multiples.

ORGANIZATIONS

National Organizations of Mothers of Twins Clubs (NOMOTC)
P.O. Box 700860
Plymouth, MI 48170-0955
877-540-2200

Representing over 475 clubs in cities all over the United States, the NOMOTC is the oldest and largest organization serving multiple-birth families today. Locate a club near you, read the latest news on multiples, and find ongoing research projects for multiples at their Web site.

Pregnancy Loss–Related Organizations

SHARE
www.NationalSHAREOffice.com
SHARE is an organization dedicated to helping you grieve the loss of your child, no matter at what point your child died. Through a monthly paper newsletter that is free for the first year, to conferences held all over, SHARE has support at heart.

Fertility-Related Resources

WEB SITES
About Infertility Guide
infertility.about.com
Infertility from diagnosis to high-tech assistance. This site includes a personal touch with lots of opportunities for loving support from others in your situation. A great place to look for cycle buddies.

BOOKS
The Everything® Getting Pregnant Book by Robin Elise Weiss
A guide to every aspect of getting pregnant, from preparing your body for pregnancy to timing your pregnancy. Even includes a section on secondary infertility and fertility treatments.

Taking Charge of Your Fertility by Toni Weschler, M.P.H.
This is an excellent manual for learning about charting your natural fertility cycles. It goes into very great detail about charting your basal body temperatures.

FERTILITY-RELATED ORGANIZATIONS
American Society for Reproductive Medicine (ASRM) (Formerly the American Fertility Society)
1209 Montgomery Highway
Birmingham, AL 35216-2809
Phone: 205-978-5000
Fax: 205-978-5005
www.asrm.org
ASRM provides patient and physician information. It also helps govern and provide guidance for fertility programs, both in training and in ethical situations. You will find great handouts on various positions from ASRM here, also included in Spanish.

Couple to Couple League—Natural Family Planning

www.ccli.org

The Couple to Couple League provides training in various locations about how to use your body's fertility signals to help you achieve pregnancy and diagnose your cycle variability. This can be used to help achieve or avoid pregnancy with great accuracy. Their Web site includes information on finding local classes.

The International Council on Infertility Information Dissemination, Inc. (INCIID)

P.O. Box 6836
Arlington, VA 22206
Phone: 703-379-9178
Fax: 703-379-1593
www.inciid.org

Great information for support purposes and information. They offer chats by professionals for the layperson on various forms of fertility questions.

RESOLVE: The National Infertility Association

1310 Broadway
Somerville, MA 02144
888-623-0744
E-mail: info@resolve.org
www.resolve.org

Primarily a support organization for persons facing various fertility issues. Leadership positions in this organization are held by professionals in the field, as well as parents.

Society for Assisted Reproductive Technology (SART)

1209 Montgomery Highway
Birmingham, AL 35216
Phone: 205-978-5000 (x109)
Fax: 205-978-5015
E-mail: jzeitz@asrm.org
www.sart.org

SART runs the statistical information processing that is used in helping you compare fertility clinic to fertility clinic. It should be consulted when trying to decide what program is right for you.

Index

Index